CL

Detox Your Body, Mind and Spirit
Betty Murray, CN, HHC, RYT

Cindy,

Live Well. Be Well. Eat Well!

LIVING WELL PUBLISHING | DALLAS, TEXAS

Living Well Publishing
An imprint of Living Well Dallas, Limited Liability Corporation
14330 Midway Road, Suite 121
Dallas TX 7544

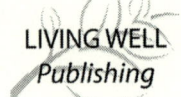

Copyright © 2013, by Betty Murray. All rights reserved.

No part of this book may be reproduced or transmitted in any form or by any means, electronic or mechanical, including photocopying, recording or by any information storage and retrieval system, without written permission from the author, except for the inclusion of brief quotations in a review.

For more information regarding special discounts for bulk purchases, please contact the publisher at 972-930-0260 or by email at info@livingwelldallas.com

A goodmedia communications, llc book.
www.goodmediacommunications.com
Cover & Book Design by goodmedia communications, llc

The text in this book is set in Gill Sans.
ISBN 10: 0-9842985-1-7
ISBN 13: 978-0-9842985-1-8
Manufactured in the United States of America

DISCLAIMER: ALL INFORMATION MATERIAL FOUND HEREIN IS PROVIDED FOR GENERAL INFORMATION PURPOSES ONLY. THE INFORMATION AND MATERIAL PROVIDED IS NOT INTENDED TO DIAGNOSE OR TREAT ANY CONDITION OR SYMPTOM AND ITS USE IS NOT INTENDED TO BE A SUBSTITUTE FOR THE MEDICAL OR PROFESSIONAL ADVICE OR DIAGNOSIS OF A PHYSICIAN OR COUNSELOR. LIVING WELL DALLAS, INC. DOES NOT WARRANT OR GUARANTEE THE QUALITY, RELIABILITY, TIMELINESS, ACCURACY OR COMPLETENESS OF ANY INFORMATION HEREIN AND THE INFORMATION IS PROVIDED WITHOUT WARRANTY, AND LIVING WELL DALLAS, INC. SPECIFICALLY DISCLAIMS ALL WARRANTIES, EITHER EXPRESSED OR IMPLIED, STATUTORY OR OTHERWISE, INCLUDING BUT NOT LIMITED TO THE IMPLIED WARRANTIES OF MERCHANTABILITY, NON-INFRINGEMENT, AND FITNESS FOR PARTICULAR PURPOSE. LIVING WELL DALLAS, INC. IS NOT RESPONSIBLE FOR ANY DIRECT, INDIRECT, SPECIAL, PUNITIVE, INCIDENTAL OR CONSEQUENTIAL DAMAGE OR ANY OTHER DAMAGES WHATSOEVER ARISING OUT OF OR IN CONNECTION WITH THE USE OF THE INFORMATION AND MATERIAL HEREIN OR IN RELIANCE ON SUCH INFORMATION OR MATERIAL, INCLUDING, WITHOUT LIMITATION, PERSONAL INJURY, WRONGFUL DEATH, OR ANY OTHER PERSONAL OR PECUNIARY LOSS, WHETHER THE ACTION IS BASED IN CONTRACT, TORT, INCLUDING NEGLIGENCE, OR OTHERWISE.

This book is dedicated to John
for his support and love.

Table of Contents

Acknowledgments 7

Foreword 8

Preface 9

Chapter 1 11
What is a Cleanse?

Chapter 2 21
The Cleanse Quick Start Guide

Chapter 3 37
    When "Healthy" Food Hurts

Chapter 4 43
    We are What We Eat

Chapter 5 77
    A Peek in the Pantry

Chapter 6 93
    Home Is Where the Food Is

Chapter 7 103
It Takes Guts

Chapter 8 113
    Digestion: A User's Guide

Chapter 9 .... **135**
    Conscious Cleansing

Chapter 10 .... **167**
    Domestic Detox

Chapter 11 .... **187**
The Dietary Cleanse

Chapter 12 .... **239**
    Coming Off Cleanse

References **251**
The Cleanse Recipes Shopping List **255**
The Cleanse Basic Recipes **259**
The Cleanse Advanced Recipes **307**

Acknowledgments

We all hope that we will someday find our calling. For me, writing this book is a culmination of a long-standing desire to put my work to paper. I have the joy of being able to do the work that I love everyday and to interact with incredible people from all over the country. Thank you everyone who has been a part of this journey with me and to those I work with everyday making a difference in people's lives.

I would especially like to thank the following people:

My dear husband John for his unwavering love and support in every adventure I want to take.

My parents, Bonnie and Carl Brenneman, for seeing my potential even when I did not.

My business partner, Jenny Bair—my consummate cheerleader! Without her enthusiasm I may have just buried my head in the sand and let this dream slide away under the to-do-list and crazy perfectionism.

Ty Daily, my right-hand woman day in, day out, without whom I would be lost.

All of the wonderful practitioners at Living Well Health & Wellness Center whose dedication to functional medicine and making a difference in people's health and well-being is an inspiration every day.

All of my friends who bring me love and laughter every day.

The creative team at goodmedia communications, llc who helped bring this book to life. Robyn Short for her keen proofreading and editing skills as well as managing the entire writing, editing, design, printing and publishing process—especially cracking the whip to get me to finish the book!

To all of my clients past, present and future—you are my greatest teachers.

To everyone who will ever purchase this book or my other books—you all have helped me get to where I am today, and where I am going tomorrow. With love and light, I thank you!

Foreword by Robyn O'Brien

The landscape of health has changed. In the face of the jaw-dropping increases in the rates of cancer, diabetes, obesity, allergies and autism, we are no longer guaranteed a long and healthy life.

The statistics are numbing. Today, it is estimated that one out of every two men and one out of every three women will develop some form of cancer in their lifetime, one out of every three children born in the year 2000 is expected to be insulin dependent by the time they reach adulthood, and 34 percent of babies are expected to be obese by nine months of age. At the same time, one out of three American children now has autism, allergies, ADHD or asthma and cancer is the leading cause of death for children.

And the toll that these conditions are taking on our health, our families, our finances and our well-being is enormous.

Epidemics don't have genetic causes, they have environmental ones. And today, some of the greatest threats to our health aren't found in our DNA, but in our food supply. With the increasing use of antibiotics, synthetic growth hormones, pesticides, and artificial colors and dyes derived from petrochemicals, our food supply has become polluted. As a result, the mac and cheese that we are feeding our families isn't the same as the mac and cheese that we ate as kids—ours didn't contain synthetic growth hormones and artificial colors linked to hyperactivity. And the hamburger that we grew up eating didn't contain the chemicals residues now found in a fast food burger.

With this compound toxicity of our food supply, the chemicals and novel ingredients now found in our food are taking their toll not only on the health of our families but also on our finances.

The United States spends more on health care than any other developed nation in the world. From obesity to allergies, we are spending an increasing amount of our incomes managing these chronic conditions, 16 cents of every dollar, while spending on average nine cents of every dollar on food.

It doesn't have to be this way. As the high price of cheap food continues to impact our health and well-being, a call to action is occurring and Betty Murray responds with *Cleanse*. With a steady hand, moral support and a book jam-packed full of vital information, *Cleanse* is an invaluable resource for those interested in restoring the health of their families. With shopping guides, candid feedback and practical solutions, *Cleanse* is a sound investment in your health and a book that will pay health dividends for a lifetime.

Preface

> *The significant problems we have cannot be solved at the same level of thinking with which we created them. - Albert Einstein*

The American public, and much of the industrialized world, is on a path of chronic, life-destroying diseases. Obesity, diabetes, cardiovascular disease and cancer—diseases of affluence and abundance are killing us. American agriculture has become big business complete with high-powered marketing campaigns designed to influence our opinions and beliefs about food and nutrition. What was once a simple and intuitive task, selecting healthy foods has become a confusing chore. Junk food and health food are manufactured and packaged to look the same. Even the most well intended consumer falls prey to the marketing ploys of the big food companies. With good nutrition being the single most important component to achieving and sustaining wellness, American consumers must have a solid working knowledge of how food affects the body both positively and negatively.

Just as a symphony requires the collaboration and coordinated timing of strings, horns and percussion, the body requires a similar synchronicity of food, environment, body systems and chemical processes all working in a coordinated effort. And, just as one musician playing off-key or missing a beat will disrupt the harmony and beauty of the symphony, so does poor nutrition or toxic environmental inputs disrupt the harmony of wellness.

As a nutritionist and owner of Living Well Health & Wellness Center, an integrative medical center on the leading edge of applied functional medicine and clinical nutrition, I have had the unique opportunity of assisting thousands of people in achieving a better level of health and wellness. Nutritional therapy is the foundation of wellness. At Living Well Health & Wellness Center, we solve tough problems for people who have not been able to find help with traditional medical approaches. This experience makes it easier for me to understand and help people who have resigned themselves to the belief that it is normal to feel a general malaise.

The purpose of this book is to help people understand that feeling bad is not normal, having a spare tire is not normal and falling apart as we age is not normal. Our bodies are designed for greatness. This book will help people obtain a healthy lifestyle by reducing nagging physical symptoms, teaching people how to naturally cleanse the body, and by providing a healthy and effective weight loss method and create a permanent lifestyle change using the principles found in this book.

I designed The Cleanse Program™, also a three-week workshop series, as a means of bringing my natural foods-based program to large audiences. Prior to this program, only clients who were able to meet with me one-on-one had access to this information. Soon after launching The Cleanse Program workshop series, I began receiving requests from friends of participants and from other health centers requesting that I bring The Cleanse Program to their area or center. As the demand for The Cleanse Program continued to grow and participants began coming back for repeat workshops, I realized the need for a comprehensive guide that people could refer to long after the workshop series ended. *Cleanse: Detox Your Body, Mind and Spirit* offers easy to implement, natural processes developed in The Cleanse Program that anyone can do to cleanse the body, reduce negative physical symptoms and improve health. This book lays the foundation for why cleansing is important and provides a thorough explanation of how the body systems function. People who are serious about strengthening their overall health must be committed to ongoing self-improvement and should avail themselves of many resources. *Cleanse* is the first step in this process.

My wish is that this book brings readers the knowledge and usable health information necessary to live healthier and happier lives now and in the future.

Betty Murray

What is a Cleanse?

> *Keeping your body healthy is an expression of gratitude to the whole cosmos—the trees, the clouds, everything.*
> *- Thich Nhat Hanh*

Today you may have pulled yourself out of bed with a stuffy nose, congestion or a general sense of exhaustion, fatigue and ache. You may have lost that loving feeling (libido), gained weight around the middle and decided you are destined to wear "mom jeans" from here on out. You may have resigned yourself to the fact you are getting older, the pollen where you live is your dreaded enemy and that your work, lack of restful sleep or too many calories without enough exercise are the cause for your body's downfall and malaise. You may decide that taking an antihistamine for the congestion is the answer to your allergies, downing significant amounts coffee gives you just enough energy, and your passion is simply gone. You hobble off to work thinking that this is what life is like at your age.

I am here to tell you that your life is not designed to be on a slow decline until you eventually peter out and fall in the grave. We are designed to live a healthy, productive and energetic life throughout our years. The symptoms many people live with and assume are natural effects of aging are merely the body's reactions to its environment. The "environment" is everything we put into our bodies, everything we expose our bodies to, our thoughts as well as our emotional responses to those thoughts.

By changing our environment, we can change our physical bodies. Fortunately, we have the power to control our environment and regain, or maintain, a state of wellness.

We have been taught to believe that our diagnosed symptoms of "dis-ease" are actual diseases that require drugs to suppress them. I believe, and I am not alone in this belief, that symptoms are just reminders that something is out of balance in the body. Regardless of the diagnosis, if the root cause can be found and brought into balance, then wellness (reduction or elimination of symptoms) may be restored.

People often experience several symptoms, which means there may be several underlying imbalances that are synergistically contributing to the dis-ease. Many people come to me for assistance with one concern such as fatigue or weight gain; however, most of my clients have let their condition progress to the point that they now have multiple causes for their complaints. These complaints require a holistic approach to get to the root problem because correcting one issue does not result in 100 percent reduction of the symptoms.

Dr. Sidney Baker has a great analogy that I often borrow to make this point: The "Tack Rule." If you sit on one tack, removing it makes you feel a whole lot better. But if you sit on two tacks, removing one tack does not result in a 50 percent improvement. You may have a headache (tack) for which you take aspirin (to suppress the headache symptom) only to find that you get the headache again after the aspirin wears off. Often, the headache is not the root problem; it is merely one of the tacks you have been sitting on.

So, what kind of symptoms might you be living with that have a direct correlation to the foods you eat, the cleaning products you use or the environment in which you live and work? Do you suffer from any of the following?

- Acne & blemishes
- Allergies
- Arthritis and joint pain
- Asthma
- Bladder disorders
- Blood sugar disorders
- Circulatory problems
- Chronic digestive issues
- Craving sweets and/or salty foods
- Eczema and rashes
- Edema (swelling)
- Fatigue
- Food allergies
- Hair loss
- Hair/skin & nail disorders
- Inflammation
- Kidney disease
- Low libido
- Migraines & headaches
- PMS/ PMDD & hormonal imbalances
- Weight gain and/or inability to lose weight

If you are like most of my clients, you are so accustomed to feeling poorly that you either: 1) fail to recognize how bad you feel until you feel better while on The Cleanse Program; or, 2) you feel bad and have no idea if what you eat may be contributing.

Do you have any of these chronic issues? By chronic, I mean consistently occurring and resulting in a downgrading of your health and well-being. Chronic does not necessarily mean a chronic disease, although this too can be addressed in the same manner. Chronic conditions have two main causes: 1) Some environmental input is causing irritation or is undesirable to the body such as allergies or toxins; and 2) the lack of, or need for, a particular substance (deficiency) the body is not getting or not getting enough of.

The Cleanse Program is designed to remove the most common culprits (tacks) that cause irritation to the body and introduce many of the nutrients and foods that may be missing, or in short supply in your diet such as green leafy foods or water to assist the body in achieving balance. The Cleanse Program is not a panacea or a cure for anything. The program is designed to be a tool for you to use to be able to determine if what you eat and use on your body and in your home may be interfering with your quality of living.

If, through The Cleanse Program, you find that the foods you previously ate interfered with your health, you will know what to eliminate from your diet and/or lifestyle. Through this program you will gain the knowledge and power to choose foods that either detract or add to your health. Obviously a diet of fast, processed foods is generally not healthy and leads to undesirable symptoms, but sometimes even healthy foods are not healthy for everyone.

The Cleanse Program is an eating program that uses foods to achieve the following: improve the functions of the body, particularly digestion; remove potential allergens and irritants; and introduce a whole foods approach to daily living. I designed The Cleanse Program to be easily accessible and useful for most people, even people who travel frequently, dine out often or have hectic schedules.

Every commercial cleanse you read about is different. Some cleanse programs focus on weight loss, others on decreasing allergy symptoms, killing parasites or cleansing the liver and gallbladder. Some cleanses can take days, others take weeks or months. For the sake of simplicity, most cleanses can be classified as either dietary cleanses or supplemental cleanses that require heroic dietary changes such as juicing only or buying and consuming significant amounts of supplements.

I believe that cleansing can be subtler without losing effectiveness. I also believe that in order for a cleanse to be effective it must be easy to implement for a period of time. It does no good to juice and pop pills on the weekend trying to cleanse the liver only to go off the cleanse when you go back to work (i.e., downing coffee and eating fast food).

I am also leery of cleanses designed to affect the liver detoxification process without testing a person's liver detoxification functions. Many of the boxed and processed cleanse products contain several herbs and nutrients that speed up or slow down the steps the liver takes to detox. After years of testing people in my practice, I found that you can never be sure about liver function until you test it. And, if you do not test prior to implementing a liver detox, it is very likely you will experience unpleasant and potentially severe side effects.

Additionally, supplements designed to detox the liver without dietary adjustments are generally not effective because the human body is an integrated system within which all of the parts work synergistically. Material that is cleansed from the liver will exit from the body through the skin, kidneys and/or colon. If the colon, kidneys and/or skin are not operating at peak efficiency, a liver cleanse can do more harm than good as toxins expelled from the liver circulate and are reabsorbed rather than flushed from the body.

The Cleanse Program is designed to accomplish the following:

- Remove the top foods that may be contributing to unhealthy symptoms.
- Remove environmental toxins.
- Introduce foods that are whole and unprocessed.
- Improve the body's digestive functions including all digestive organs.
- Provide lifestyle tips for improving the body-mind-spirit connection.

UNDERSTANDING THE CLEANSE PROCESS

Imagine you have 20 guests in your home for a Super Bowl party. The house looks clean, but you may have hidden clutter in the office or closets. Halfway through the party, the plumbing becomes clogged. It does not take long for the plumbing to backup and cause a significant problem. Quite possibly the mess will overflow from the bathroom into the other rooms in the house, maybe the office or closets where you have hidden additional clutter. Now you have a toxic mess (plumbing leak) overrunning your house (body) and even mixing with, and further polluting, your hidden mess in the closets. Ultimately the party ends, your house is a complete wreck, and you now have a toxic situation on your hands—the plumbing problem combined with toxic clutter still hiding in your closets.

Cleansing the liver without addressing the digestive tract will have the same effect. Now let's make this analogy work for the body. Our bodies have a sophisticated plumbing system (digestive tract and elimination organs) that flushes the system regularly to prevent nasty toxins and waste from overrunning the body. Our fat cells are the storage sites (office and closets) where our bodies hide our unmentionable trash until it can clean it out later through the detoxification process in the liver. If the digestive tract, specifically the elimination organs (plumbing), become clogged, the backup will be significantly unpleasant. Toxins will seep into the other organs (rooms). The fat cells (office and closets) will begin to dump toxins into the liver for processing or filtering.

To complete the analogy, the house is spinning out of control with the backed up plumbing (the digestive tract) and hidden, toxic, clutter (toxic organs), and you don't know what to address first—the backed up plumbing or the overflowing toxic trash—as they are both destroying your house (your body). Ultimately, the clogged plumbing (digestive tract) must be repaired first and then a massive cleanup on the toxic trash must take place (a cleansing of the organs).

For this reason, an effective cleanse regimen should get the digestive tract, colon, kidneys and skin working optimally before addressing the liver detoxification process so that toxins are properly removed from the body and do not result in illness or negative reactions during the cleanse. If a cleanse it too hard on the body, negative reactions such as flu-like symptoms, headaches, gastrointestinal distress and other uncomfortable symptoms may occur. An effective cleanse should not be a "no pain, no gain" program.

The detoxification process in the body, or cleansing of the body, is an incredibly important and necessary function. Over 75 percent of the nutrition (vitamins, minerals, amino acids, etc.) a person consumes through food is used for the detoxification process. If we eat foods that are nutrient poor, the liver will be forced to work overtime and will not able to detoxify optimally.

ENVIRONMENTAL TOXINS

Dietary inputs are only one way in which the body can become toxic. We all encounter innumerable toxins in our daily lives. Pollution is everywhere. Pollutants are in the air we breathe, the food we eat and the water we drink.

Toxins are in the detergent most of us use to wash our bodies, our food, our homes and our laundry. Chemicals comprise the pharmaceutical drugs we take. Chemicals are infused in our homes via carpet, paint, fabric and plastics as well as in our electronic gadgets. Simply stated, the modern world is a highly toxic world. However, for better or worse, it is the world in which we live.

If you are not yet disturbed, read on. A study released by the Centers for Disease Control found that people are still carrying traces of dangerous chemicals banned 25–30 years ago. A study published by *British Medical Journal* estimated that 75 percent of most cancers are caused by environmental and lifestyle factors, including exposure to chemicals. Columbia University's School of Public Health published a report estimating that 95 percent of cancer is caused by diet and environmental toxicity.

Consider this ...

- An estimated 100,000 chemicals are produced in North America alone.
- There are over 4,000 chemicals routinely added to our food.
- More than 10,000 chemical solvents, emulsifiers and preservatives are used in food processing.
- Recent studies indicate that 4,000 new chemicals are introduced into the environment each year.

Where do all of these chemicals end up? They are absorbed into our groundwater, rivers, lakes and oceans, spewed into our air, and added, quite intentionally, to our food supply. All of these pollutants—chemicals and toxins—eventual end up in our bodies through oral consumption, inhalation or via contact with our skin. These toxins build up a residue in our bodies and greatly contribute to our ability, or lack thereof, to have healthy metabolic rates and healthy immune functions. Most health practitioners will agree that just about every disease and health problem can be directly or indirectly traced back to toxicity in the body. This toxicity manifests as congestion, chronic digestive disorders, migraines, PMS/PMDD and hormonal imbalances, inflammation, fatigue, weight gain, chronic pain and illness. Never before has cleansing the body of these toxins been more important. A cleanse can bring relief of chronic pain, swelling, fatigue, allergies, attention deficit and improve virtually all aspects of mental and physical health.

While one may think of pollutants as a problem of the modern world, the idea of cleansing the body is not new. As a matter of fact, long before it became part of a healthy lifestyle, cleansing was a regular part of all spiritual practices.

All religions incorporate some level of fasting or cleansing of the body for purity. The word breakfast comes from the tradition of breaking a fast. Most traditional cleanses work with the fasting model—consuming no food for a period of time. A cleanse or fast is often the preparation for a spiritual practice.

There are several key components to The Cleanse Program. The first is to ensure that you are receiving optimal nutritional intake of both macro and micronutrients. The second component is to increase dietary fiber and hydration, both of which will assist in flushing the toxins out of the body. The third component is to create an acid alkaline balance through dietary changes. The fourth component is a cleansing of the digestive system, specifically the liver and lymph, which is achieved as a result of all of the above actions.

WHAT TO EXPECT ON THE CLEANSE PROGRAM

To reap the full benefits of this program, it is necessary to change more than what goes into your mouth. You must make changes in everything that goes into your life. A truly holistic cleanse will create a shift towards a cleaner environment, healthier interpersonal relationships, as well as a greater sense of emotional well-being.

While most people feel dramatically better, even lighter and happier, during and after the cleanse, that is not the case for all people. The intensity of the cleansing processes releases more than just physical toxins. A cleanse should, and most likely will, release toxic emotions resulting in a shift in how you experience your own sense of self, as well as how you experience your important relationships.

You may experience bouts of anger, sadness and other strong emotions during a cleanse. If you should have this experience, rest assured that this is ultimately a good experience—this is the process of releasing the toxic accumulation that has been stored in your body. Exercises and ideas to help with the mental and emotional side of cleansing are included in this book.

Are you ready? Let's go!

Your Total Toxic Burden Assessment

Let's see how toxic you are! This assessment will help you determine many of the areas of your diet and lifestyle that may be contributing to your toxic burden.

Please take this assessment and consider all of your responses that have a (-) answer. These areas may be contributing to an increased risk of a toxic overload.

Are you over weight or do you tend to over eat at meals?

☐ Yes (-1)   ☐ No (+1)

Do you experience GI complaints such as constipation, gas or diarrhea?

☐ Yes (-1)   ☐ No (+1)

Do you consume more than four ounces of alcohol each day?

☐ Yes (-1)   ☐ No (+1)

Do you regularly use over-the-counter medications (e.g., painkillers and antihistamines)?

☐ Yes (-1)   ☐ No (+1)

Are you taking any prescribed medications on a daily basis?

☐ Yes (-1)   ☐ No (+1)

How many fast food meals do you eat each week?

☐ (+1) None   ☐ (-2) 1-2 meals   ☐ (-4) 3 or more meals

Do you consume artificial sweeteners such as aspartame, sucralose (Splenda) or saccharin?

☐ Yes (-1)   ☐ No (+1)

Do you eat foods that are artificially colored?

☐ Yes (-1)   ☐ No (+1)

What time of day do you typically eat refined carbohydrates or sugar?

☐ Never (+1) ☐ Morning (-1) ☐ Afternoon (-1)
☐ Evening (-2) ☐ Afternoon & Evening (-3) ☐ All day (-4)

How many different colors of vegetables & fruits do you eat in a day?

☐ 0-1 colors (-1) ☐ 2-4 colors (+1) ☐ 5-7 colors (+3)

Do you drink more than one 8-ounce cup of coffee?

☐ Yes (-1) ☐ No (+1)

How many 8-ounce glasses of filtered, spring or mineral water do you drink every day?

☐ (-3) None ☐ (+1) 1-3 glasses
☐ (+2) 4-7 glasses ☐ (+3) 7-10 glasses

Do you cook or re-heat foods in plastic containers in the microwave?

☐ Yes (-1) ☐ No (+1)

Do you use pesticides in your house or on your lawn?

☐ Yes (-1) ☐ No (+1)

Do you expose yourself to toxins such as traditional household cleaners?

☐ Yes (-1) ☐ No (+1)

Add up your responses, and refer to the scoring below:

_____ Total Score

If your score is more than -5 on the total score, you may want to consider the questions where you had a negative (-) score. These are areas where changing your habits could have a significant impact on your health.

Disclaimer: This assessment is not intended to be a substitute for a professionally conducted laboratory screening and assessment. This assessment should be used as a self-guided tool to identify areas in which making changes to your diet and lifestyle may improve your well-being

2
The Cleanse Quick Start Guide

The greatest wealth is health. - Virgil

LYNNE ANNE SMITH, TESTIMONIAL

I started The Cleanse Program because I thought that I would want to do a fast with juicing to jumpstart a weight loss regimen. I had heard of juice cleanses from friends. When I started the class, I had no idea that I could really cleanse my body without taking extreme measures such as juicing for days on end. I was actually relieved. I had primed myself for starving and having to buy tons of vegetables and drinking stuff that tasted like grass. The Cleanse Program was so easy, and I was very happy that I could eat real food.

I was surprised to gain a full understanding of how digestion works and especially how the liver utilizes nutrition. I had no idea that food played such an important role in how we feel. Knowing, as Betty Murray said, the "what" and "why" really made a huge difference for me in terms of keeping me motivated to stay on the program.

During The Cleanse Program, I did go through some withdrawal from Diet Coke and other caffeinated drinks, but it only lasted a few days. I was surprised to realize how much more energy I had after eliminating caffeine from my diet.

I also found that I started to lose inches even before the number on my scale moved down. During The Cleanse Program I had regular bowel movements for the first time in my life. A doctor once told me that going to the bathroom once every few days was normal. I know better now. I discovered that eggs and dairy was the culprit to my slow digestion.

On this The Cleanse Program, I learned to master my emotional eating triggers. I have a newfound respect for food and will continue with the cleanse lifestyle.

QUICK START GUIDE

If you are ready and raring to go, you can use this quick start guide to get going right now. The Quick Start Guide will give you the nuts and bolts of The Cleanse Program. If you do not want to start without reading all of the "who," "what," "why," and "when," then skip the Quick Start Guide and move on to chapter three. A more detailed guide to The Cleanse Program can be found in chapter eleven, The Dietary Cleanse.

PLANNING

Planning is the area n in which most people trip up when trying to start new healthy habits. It is important to take the time to follow each of the steps in The Cleanse Program so that your experience is easier and more effective. Included is a three-day preparation guide, or you can create your own plan that works with your lifestyle.

TALK TO YOUR DOCTOR

Please inform your doctor any time you make changes to your diet and lifestyle. If you suffer from any illness, it is important that your doctor approves, or is aware, of any major shifts in diet, lifestyle and exercise.

If your doctor is concerned about The Cleanse Program, you can highlight the fact that The Cleanse Program contains *real* whole foods and healthy new eating habits. This is not a calorie-restriction program. You will be required to remove processed, toxic, fake and "franken-foods" such as hydrogenated oils, soda and fast foods from your diet. You will be eating only whole, nutritious and preferably organic foods.

PREPARING YOUR KITCHEN

Get your kitchen ready! If you cannot find your kitchen because of the sea of mail that has taken over the countertop, it is time to get some organization going.

You will not need any fancy kitchen gadgets such as juicers or a spiral slicer. A blender and a Crockpot® are good items to have, but are not required. A sharp set of kitchen knives, cutting board and stainless steel pots or pans will be sufficient for you to do the cleanse.

COOKWARE

You may be surprised to learn that your cookware is a serious toxin contender. The safest cookware to use is ceramic-coated, cast iron or stainless steel cookware. Pyrex glass is also safe to cook with; just let it cool completely before washing to reduce the chance of it shattering.

UNSAFE COOKWARE

Anodized, Teflon® or any other nonstick surface cookware are not safe to use. After just a few minutes on a conventional stovetop, cookware coated with Teflon and other nonstick surfaces can exceed temperatures at which the coating breaks apart and emits toxic particles into the air. Enough said! Teflon and anodized nonstick pans are bad news!

Although aluminum is not considered to be as bad as lead, it can be toxic in excessive amounts and even in small amounts if it is deposited in the brain. Aluminum toxicity can cause symptoms of colic, rickets, gastrointestinal problems, interference with the metabolism of calcium, extreme nervousness, anemia, headaches, decreased liver and kidney function, memory loss, speech problems, softening of the bones and aching muscles. Cooking with aluminum pans increases your toxic exposure, especially if you cook acidic foods such as tomato sauce. By the way, municipal water is the largest source of aluminum in the American diet.

PREPARE THE PANTRY

One of the most supportive actions you can make is to banish the enemy! If your pantry, desk drawer at work and refrigerator are full of toxic, processed foods and junk, it will make it harder to stay on the cleanse. Now, some people reading this just got a vivid picture of mutiny in the house! What will the rest of the family eat? Well, they could participate on the cleanse with you. The Cleanse Program is healthy for people of all ages. Or, you can simply remove the things that are most tempting to you. If you cannot bear to throw food out, you can donate nonperishable items to a food bank.

WHAT TO EAT?

The Cleanse Program allows for fresh, seasonal, whole foods. Most of these foods reside on the perimeter of the grocery store aisles. At the end of this book are plenty of recipes that incorporate all the foods you can eat. If you are a recipe rebel, have no fear! You can use the following list of foods, spices and cooking techniques to make your own meal creations. Just stay within the rules, and you will be right on track.

So let's get to the nuts and bolts of shopping. The following are the acceptable foods for The Cleanse Program.

Cleanse for Beginners Shopping List

Protein

- ☐ Cold water fish: salmon, halibut, cod, mackerel, tuna, sardines, anchovies
- ☐ Shellfish
- ☐ Lean chicken
- ☐ Turkey, chicken
- ☐ Lean red meats
- ☐ Lamb
- ☐ Grass fed buffalo, beef

Protein Powders

- ☐ Cleanse Detox Formula
- ☐ Rice Protein
- ☐ Hemp Protein
- ☐ Pea Protein

Fats

- ☐ Avocado
- ☐ Clarified butter
- ☐ Coconut milk or oil
- ☐ High-quality fish oil
- ☐ Flaxseed oil
- ☐ Freshly ground flaxseed meal
- ☐ Macadamia nuts
- ☐ Olive oil, olives
- ☐ Raw nuts & seeds

Non-Starchy Vegetables

- ☐ Arugula
- ☐ Asparagus
- ☐ Bamboo shoots
- ☐ Bean sprouts
- ☐ Beet greens
- ☐ Bell peppers (red, yellow, green)
- ☐ Broccoli
- ☐ Brussels sprouts
- ☐ Cabbage
- ☐ Cassava
- ☐ Cauliflower
- ☐ Celery
- ☐ Chayote fruit
- ☐ Chicory
- ☐ Chives
- ☐ Collard greens
- ☐ Coriander
- ☐ Cucumber
- ☐ Dandelion greens
- ☐ Eggplant
- ☐ Endive
- ☐ Fennel
- ☐ Garlic
- ☐ Ginger root
- ☐ Green beans
- ☐ Hearts of palm
- ☐ Jicama (raw)
- ☐ Jalapeno peppers
- ☐ Kale
- ☐ Kohlrabi
- ☐ Lettuce
- ☐ Mushrooms
- ☐ Mustard greens
- ☐ Onions
- ☐ Parsley
- ☐ Radishes
- ☐ Radicchio
- ☐ Snap beans
- ☐ Snow peas
- ☐ Shallots
- ☐ Spinach
- ☐ Spaghetti squash
- ☐ Summer squash
- ☐ Swiss chard
- ☐ Tomatoes

- ☐ Turnip greens
- ☐ Watercress

High Fiber Starchy Vegetables

- ☐ Artichokes
- ☐ Chick peas/ garbanzo beans, Aduki, Black bean
- ☐ Leeks
- ☐ French beans
- ☐ Okra
- ☐ Jerusalem Artichokes
- ☐ Pumpkin
- ☐ Squash (acorn, butternut, winter)
- ☐ Sweet potato or yam
- ☐ Turnips
- ☐ Beets
- ☐ Rutabaga
- ☐ Carrots and parsnips

Grains

- ☐ Amaranth
- ☐ Brown rice
- ☐ Buckwheat
- ☐ Millet
- ☐ Quinoa
- ☐ Wild rice

Fruits

- ☐ Apples
- ☐ Berries (blackberries, blueberries, raspberries, strawberries)
- ☐ Grapefruit
- ☐ Lemons
- ☐ Limes
- ☐ Pear

Spices

This is by no means an exhaustive list, but I included it to let you know that cleansing is not boring. Using herbs can spice up your life and increase the cleansing power of foods!

- ☐ Black pepper and white pepper
- ☐ Cayenne Pepper
- ☐ Cilantro
- ☐ Cinnamon
- ☐ Cloves
- ☐ Tunermic
- ☐ Dill
- ☐ Garlic
- ☐ Ginger Root
- ☐ Fennel
- ☐ Oregano
- ☐ Paprika
- ☐ Parsley
- ☐ Peppermint
- ☐ Rosemary
- ☐ Sage
- ☐ Cumin
- ☐ Tarragon
- ☐ Basil
- ☐ Oregano
- ☐ Lemongrass
- ☐ Sea salt

THE CLEANSE PROGRAM DAILY REGIMEN

The following three steps should be completed every day while on The Cleanse Program. Many people choose to continue with this regimen post-cleanse.

STEP 1: HYDRATION AND LYMPHATIC STIMULANT

Daily Hydration – Flushing your system and reducing sugar cravings

- Mix 2-ounces of organic, non-sweetened cranberry, pomegranate or acai juice (not from concentrate) with 32-ounces of water equaling a MINIMUM of 34-ounces. Drink this beverage throughout the day.
- Drink an additional 64-ounces of filtered or spring water at room temperature or warm with a squeeze of lemon and lime juice.
- You may drink two to four cups of herbal teas to aid in detoxification. These can count toward your regular water intake as long as they do not contain caffeine. I enjoy red clover and licorice tea.

STEP 2: GUT HEALING MORNING SMOOTHIE/PUDDING

- Take ½-cup of organic apple or pear sauce with or without cinnamon.
- Add one to three tablespoons ground flax meal.
- *Optional* - Add one tablespoon glutamine powder for extra healing.
- Mix all ingredients together and then enjoy as a pudding or use the mixed ingredients as a base for a morning smoothie with Cleanse Detox Formula added.

STEP 3: PUTTING OUT THE INFLAMMATION FIRE

- Take one tablespoon of flax oil either in your Gut Healing Smoothie, or use it to make salad dressings. You can also just take a tablespoon a day.

THE CLEANSE PROGRAM FOODS

Non-Vegetarians

- VEGETABLES! Increase vegetables, especially leafy greens. Eat at least five to seven servings a day (1-cup raw or ½-Cup cooked).
- Eat lean proteins (fish, fowl, buffalo, game and lean red meat).
- Eat vegetable soups for lunch or dinner to rest digestion (great for lunch).
- Supplement protein intake with Cleanse Detox Formula or rice protein shakes made with berries. Do not use whey, casein, egg or soy protein.
- Increase omega-3 fat intake by adding flax oil daily on steamed vegetables.
- Eat tree nuts (walnuts, almonds and pecans) to increase good fats.
- Eat an apple a day for additional fiber.
- You may need to eat five to six small meals throughout the day. If you have blood sugar management issues, you will probably get hungry more frequently. If you do not have blood sugar issues, you may find three to four meals are perfect for you.
- You may have one servings (½-cup) of brown rice, millet, quinoa or amaranth grain in its natural cooked form each day. Over the course of the cleanse we will limit the grain intake and use vegetables instead.
- Root vegetables such as beets, carrots, turnips and rutabaga are all great choices for vegetable forms of starch.
- Drink green, white or black tea to wean yourself off coffee and other stimulants.
- Drink two to four herbal teas a day to improve the detoxification process.
- Use stevia or xylitol to sweeten foods.

Vegetarians

- VEGETABLES! Increase vegetables, especially leafy greens. Eat at least five to seven servings a day (1-cup raw or ½-cup cooked).
- Supplement protein with The Cleanse Functional Food, rice or hemp protein powder. Do not use soy, whey, egg or casein powders.
- Eat vegetable soups for lunch or dinner to rest digestion (great for lunch).

- Supplement protein intake with rice protein shakes made with berries.
- Increase omega-3 fat intake by adding flax oil daily on steamed vegetables.
- Eat tree nuts (walnuts, almonds and pecans) to increase good fats.
- Eat an apple a day for additional fiber.
- You may need to eat five to six small meals throughout the day. If you have blood sugar management issues, you will probably get hungry more frequently. If you do not have blood sugar issues, you may find three to four meals are perfect for you.
- You may have one to two servings (½-cup) of brown rice, millet, quinoa or amaranth grain in its natural cooked form a day. Try and limit the grain intake and use vegetables instead.
- Root vegetables such as beets, carrots, turnips and rutabaga are all great choices for vegetable forms of starch.
- Eat one to two ½-cup servings of black beans, garbanzo beans, lentils, black-eyed peas, adzuki beans, aduki beans, field peas and green peas for protein.
- Drink green, white or black tea to wean yourself off coffee and other stimulants.
- Drink one to four cups herbal teas each day to improve the detoxification process.
- Use stevia, or xylitol to sweeten foods.

FOODS NOT ALLOWED ON THE CLEANSE PROGRAM

You will be removing all of the top allergen foods: soy, wheat, dairy, sugar, orange and high sugar fruits, yeast, peanuts, eggs and corn.

- No dairy foods: milk, cheese, yogurt, ice cream and cream.
- No high-glycemic sugar fruits: pineapple, banana, melons and mangos.
- No wheat or gluten-containing grains: wheat, cereal, wheat berries, spelt, bulgur, rye grains, pasta, crackers, cereals and breads.
- No peanuts: Peanuts are not actually nuts.
- No soy foods: tofu, tempeh and soy sauce.

- No orange or tangerine citrus.
- No oatmeal as it is usually processed in plants where wheat is also processed.
- No eggs or foods containing eggs.

Remove Sugar, Alcohol, Caffeine and Toxic Chemicals

Sugar depletes the body of minerals. In order to be broken down, the body will leech minerals from bones and tissues.

Alcohol must be cleansed by the liver and causes substantial damage to the liver tissue. It preferentially gets absorbed and converted to sugar over food and goes straight to the belly in the form of fat.

Fake sweeteners such as Aspartame, Saccharin and Sucralose are neurotoxins that damage the nervous system and lead to mood, cognitive and behavioral disorders.

Caffeine is a psychoactive drug that can cause damage to the central nervous system, and leads to addiction and adrenal stress.

Remove Gluten-Containing Grains

Wheat, rye, splet, barley and tricale have a breakdown protein component called gliadin that is indigestible by human. In a substantial part of the population, gliadin causes an immune response that can damage the small intestines causing intestinal permeability, malnourishment and a host of other disorders leading to digestive complaints, IBS, neurological and behavioral issues, mood disorders, joint pain as well as weight loss resistance.

Remove all forms of Dairy

Many people are sensitive to the casein found in dairy (cheese), as well as whey protein. Casein sensitivities play a heavy role in mood and cognitive disorders, digestive and allergy disorders. Dairy causes excess mucus and exacerbates allergies and skin breakouts

Remove Highly Acidic Beans

Beans contain a harmful toxin (phytohemagglutinin) that must be removed, usually by soaking and cooking as well as having a high lectin content which can activate our immune system. Many beans are highly acidic and difficult to digest. All beans contain oligosaccharides which is indigestible by humans because we do not make this enzymes.

For this reason, a good balance of intestinal bacteria is needed to digest beans since we are already at a deficit with insufficient enzymes. People with gas and bloating after eating beans often have an out of balance ecosystem of gut bacteria resulting in the improper fermentation of the sugars in beans in the large intestines by the bacteria.

The hardest beans to digest are kidney, pinto and navy beans. On The Cleanse Program we remove all beans except garbanzo/chickpeas, aduki and black beans.

Remove Soy Foods

Soy is one of the top five food allergens. Almost all packaged foods contain soy isolates. Soy contains a natural chemical that mimics estrogen, the female sex hormone and can alter estrogen levels in a human body. Soy is also difficult to digest and can cause a host of digestive issues. Only after fermentation for some time, or extensive processing, are the beans suitable for digestion.

Remove All Forms of Yeast, Fermented Foods and Fungus

Yeast in the diet increases the yeast overload often found in an out of balance gut, and a yeast overgrowth may play a significant role in many disease states and symptoms. Yeast in the gut can cause sugar cravings, digestive issues and mood changes. Yeast foods can activate the immune system and be the cause of digestive complaints, specifically brewer's and baker's yeast. Almost all packaged foods contain yeast or yeast derivatives.

Remove all vinegars except white distilled, ume plum vinegar and apple cider vinegar. These vinegars do not contain yeast or yeast by-products.

Remove Corn

Almost all packaged foods contain corn or a corn derivative. Corn may play a role in the development of asthma, chronic bronchitis and sinus infections as well as significantly activate the immune system causing allergic reactions. Corn, like much of the above list, is ubiquitous in processed foods.

Many of the symptoms of a corn sensitivity mimic the symptoms of sensitivity to other foods such as migraine headaches, asthma attacks, digestive complaints, asthma and/or shortness-of-breath.

Remove Oranges and Citrus

Citrus fruit is one of the top food allergies, especially oranges, pineapple and tangerines. Citrus fruit can cause digestive distress and other digestive complaints. Many have trouble digesting the pulp, which can lead to rather unpleasant diarrhea. Citrus foods can exacerbate acid reflux, ulcers or other sourness sensitivities. Citrus foods cause problems for people with Crohn's, IBD and IBS. It can also be a culprit in rashes on the skin around the lips or sores inside the mouth.

Remove Anything Processed

Processing—making a whole food into a processed food—destroys nutrients in the foods, reduces the fiber content and renders it useless calories in most cases. The milling, refining and stripping techniques used to process foods deplete them of their nutritive value. Oftentimes the processed food is so depleted of nutrients that the food must then be fortified so it will not cause nutrient deficiencies such as beriberi.

Breads, crackers, cereals, chips and pasta are all processed. If it comes in a box or bag, you will not be eating it on The Cleanse Program.

3-DAY COUNTDOWN

Now that you know what to buy, let's get a timeline together. Planning is where most people derail on the path to health and wellness. So do not skip this step, as it is vital to your success.

Go through the recipes in the back of the book to determine what meals you want make. You do not have to use the recipes included, but they have been crafted to remove all of the items not on The Cleanse Program without sacrificing taste.

I always start The Cleanse Program on a Sunday, which gives me a chance to use the weekend as prep days one and two. This schedule also allows me to get the first day under my belt before the workweek starts. Choose when you want to start based on your own lifestyle and schedule.

Prep Day 1

Reduce coffee consumption. You may go half caffeine-free or substitute green tea for coffee. This is also the day to make a conscious step towards reducing sugar consumption.

Shop for the following items:
- Unsweetened pomegranate, black cherry, cranberry or acai juice
- Stevia and xylitol sweeteners
- Filtered or bottled water
- Lemons and limes
- Spices and fresh herbs
  - Variety of vegetables: green leafy, cabbage, peppers, summer squash,
  - Tubers: sweet potatoes, beets, yams, carrots, red potatoes (no baking or russet).
- Cruciferous vegetables: broccoli, cabbage, cauliflower
- Flavoring vegetables: Onions, garlic, celery, cilantro, parsley
- Good Fats: Coconut Oil, Olive oil, avocado or walnut oil
- Flax oil (in the refrigerated section of most health food stores)
- Organic fish, chicken and turkey
- Brown rice, quinoa, amaranth, buckwheat and millet grain
- Almond or cashew butter
- Unsweetened almond milk (unless allergic to almonds), rice, coconut or hemp milk (found in the dairy section of the grocery store). Choose from the following brands: Almond Breeze, Pacific and Hemp Bliss, respectively.

Quality nutritional supplements are not easy to find. Most of the industry is unregulated, and therefore, supplements can be filled with less than quality fillers and chemicals. I have sourced what I believe to be the best rice protein powder supplemental food, which is the most hypo-allergenic of all sources. You are not required to use Cleanse Detox Formula; however, it will save you time and effort in finding quality choices. Purchase Cleanse Detox Formula at www.CleanseTheBook.com.

THE CLEANSE PROGRAM FOOD

If you choose to shop on your own, you want to select a rice, pea, hemp or as a last resort, a whey protein powder. For the fiber, you may buy flax meal or flax seed as a fiber source. If you buy the seed, you will need to grind it in a coffee grinder to make the seed usable.

Prep Day 2

Day two should be a big preparation day. Please take this time to get your kitchen, and your life, in order.

- Make a few jugs of unsweetened cranberry, pomegranate juice or acai and water combination.
- Grind a portion of the flax seed and store in an air-tight container in the refrigerator.
- Clean vegetables for your meals throughout the week.
  - Green leafy
  - Tubers: sweet potatoes, beets, yams, carrots, etc.
  - Cruciferous vegetables: broccoli, cabbage, cauliflower
  - Flavoring vegetables: onions, garlic, celery, cilantro, parsley
- Pre-bake several protein choices for lunches and dinner.
- Cook several servings of grains.
- Prepare a soup recipe for quick snacks or meals.

You are now ready to go!

SAMPLE DAY ON THE CLEANSE PROGRAM

You do not have to follow this exact guideline. I find spreading the water and juice mixture throughout the day is better than trying to chug it all late at night. Heed that warning or may spend a lot of time in the bathroom at night. But that is okay. Remember that's how your body eliminates waste.

Non-Vegetarian

- 6 am: 8-ounces of water with lime
- 6:15 am: 1 serving of Gut Healing Pudding with Flax and L-Glutamine
- 6:30 am: 8-ounces of pomegranate-water while exercising
- 6:30 –7 am: Exercise
- 7 am: 16-ounces of water with lime
- 8 am: Cleanse Detox Formula shake, vegetable stir-fry with broccoli, tomato, peppers and salsa, digestive enzyme with 8-ounces of water

- 9 am: 8-ounces of pomegranate-water plus multivitamin and fish oil
- 10 am: 8-ounces of licorice tea
- 11 am: 8-ounces of water with lime
- 12 pm: Thai pumpkin soup and steamed spinach with flax oil as a dressing and a digestive enzyme
- 1 pm: 8-ounces of pomegranate-water
- 3 pm: 2 tablespoons of hummus with cut red pepper as a dipper with 8-ounces of water with lime
- 5 pm: Red clover tea
- 6 pm: 10-ounces of pomegranate-water
- 6:20 pm: Poached chicken breast with a sweet potato baked (fist-sized) and a salad with lemon and olive oil, and digestive enzyme with 8-ounces of water with lemon
- 8 pm: 8-ounces of water with lime
- 10 pm/Bedtime: 8-ounces of chamomile tea

Vegetarian

- 6 am: 8-ounces of water with lime
- 6:15 am: 1-serving of Gut Healing Pudding with Flax and L-Glutamine
- 6:30 am: 16-ounces of pomegranate-water while exercising
- 6:30–7 am: Exercise
- 7 am: 8-ounces of water with lime
- 8 am: Almond milk, almond butter and The Cleanse Functional Food
- 9 am: 8-ounces of pomegranate-water, multivitamin and flax oil
- 10 am: Cinnamon baked butternut squash with 8-ounces of red clover tea
- 11 am: 16-ounces of water with lime
- 12 pm: Thai pumpkin soup and steamed spinach with flax oil as a dressing and a digestive enzyme
- 1 pm: 8-ounces of pomegranate-water
- 3 pm: 1 tablespoon of hummus with cut red pepper as a dipper

- 5 pm: 16-ounces of water with lime
- 6 pm: Zesty quinoa with broccoli & cashews with a cup of lentil soup and a digestive enzyme with 8-ounces of pomegranate-water
- 8 pm: 8-ounces of water with lime
- 8:30 pm: Apple with almond butter
- 10 pm/Bedtime: 8-ounces of chamomile tea

EXTRA MEASURES TO INCREASE CLEANSING

- Use the recipes for blended soups and blended vegetable shakes to replace at least one meal a day or use as a snack.
- Increase fiber intake by sprinkling flax meal on steamed vegetables.
- Add fish oil, a digestive enzymes and herbal teas to improve digestion.
- Add a serving of powdered greens to your water with lime for extra antioxidants.
- Add regular, sweaty exercise (walk, yoga) or saunas to your daily regimen to improve toxin removal.

Now that you have started, you should continue reading the rest of the book. The power is often not in the "what" but in the "why." This book will help you understand why our bodies become toxic, why that is so dangerous to our health and how we can reverse the damage caused by the toxins.

3
When "Healthy" Food Hurts

> *One man's meat is another man's poison.*
> *- Unknown*

ELYSE GIBSON, TESTIMONIAL

A friend encouraged me to take The Cleanse Program workshop with her. I felt that I was already healthy but might benefit by some weight loss after the holiday season. I was not prepared for the results I experienced.

I experienced no withdrawal symptoms or feelings of hunger as I ate A LOT of the "right" foods. The three weeks of The Cleanse Program were relatively easy—I liked the food, I was never hungry, and had no real cravings. The most difficult aspect was the time it took to shop and prepare my meals. The guidance and recipes were simple, all I had to do was to get to the store and do a little planning.

Somewhere in the middle of The Cleanse Program I forgot to use my inhaler that I needed at night to breathe easy. Surprisingly, at the end of three weeks, I realized I no longer needed my prescription allergy inhaler medicine that I had been taking two times a day for the past fifteen years. This was a HUGE benefit. I had no idea that diet could affect my breathing to this extent. My doctor was equally surprised. I realized that wheat and dairy were the foods leading to my asthma symptoms. As long as I did not eat wheat, and to a lesser extent dairy, I had no need for inhalers or allergy medications.

The weight loss was an exceptionally pleasant additional benefit. I stayed on The Cleanse Program for six months eating more food and more variety than I ever had before. In that six months, I continued to drop weight and got down to the weight I was when I got married. I have stabilized at that weight with little to no effort. I have continued to use what I have learned, and it has been three wonderful years of being prescription medicine free and looking and feeling great.

Not all foods, even foods typically deemed to be healthy, are good for everyone. Sometimes even healthy food hurts. Our immune system may respond to any food when eaten in several different ways. These different immune responses can go from the extreme of anaphylaxis (inability to breathe) to chronic headaches, acne and weight gain. This chapter explains the three most common immune responses triggered by foods.

An allergen is that which causes us to have an abnormal immunological response. When we have an allergic response to a particular item, we are generally responding to a particular protein molecule that is a component of the food. For instance, gluten is a protein molecule that is part of the wheat seed that many people react to.

An allergen is detected by the immune system B cells. Think of B cells as club bouncers. These are specialized immune cells capable of producing antibodies. Just like allergens, antibodies are protein molecules, but antibodies have the capacity to neutralize allergens. Every B cell produces its own, specific antibody, depending on the type of intruder it is responding to. The B-cell bouncer responds in varying degrees based on the threat level.

There are five main categories of antibodies (IgE, IgG, IgA, IgM and IgD) that the body releases under different circumstances such as fighting off various infections or ridding the body of items causing irritation. In the case of classic allergies, the body produces the antibody immunoglobulin E (IgE).

IGE-MEDIATED RESPONSE: CLASSIC ALLERGY

Usually, antibodies will bind directly to the appropriate damaging substance neutralizing it. However, IgE deviates from this common behavior and attaches a portion of its body to mast cells. The other side holds on to the offending allergen. This action signals the mast cells to begin to disintegrate, thereby releasing histamine.

Histamine is a chemical substance and neurotransmitter responsible for a great number of complaints that may arise during allergic reactions: muscle cramps, redness and swelling of mucous membranes, runny noses and itchy eyes.

IgE-mediated allergic reactions can occur under a variety of circumstances. For instance, inhaling certain substances, such as grass pollen, house dust or eating a peanut if you are allergic may cause an allergic response. Classic allergies typically bring on complaints very rapidly upon contact with the allergen. Complaints may vary from a runny nose, sinusitis, earache or runny eyes to itching of the skin, eczema and shortness of breath.

Most people know if they have a significant IgE-mediated allergy to a food. Usually this is found by accident as the result of eating the offending food and breaking out in hives or having difficulty breathing. Airborne and seasonal allergies are types of IgE-mediated immune responses.

IGG-MEDIATED RESPONSE: SENSITIVITY

Sometimes foods and other environmental exposures can bring on symptoms of IgG-mediated sensitivity. IgG antibodies are produced when the immune system B cells come in contact with the offending item, in this case, food. These antibodies are the slowly occurring variety that do not appear in the blood until three to 48 hours after exposure to an offending food or substance. IgG responses can be dose specific and often very hard to determine due to the long lead time between ingestion and the onset of symptoms.

Additionally, IgG responses have a compounding affect, meaning the immune response can be heightened if you are eating multiple offending foods. There is a synergistic affect between the multiple foods. IgG-mediated responses also can exacerbate IgE responses as well. For instance, someone with an IgG response to milk may experience greater IgE symptoms to ragweed if they consume milk regularly during the ragweed season.

Here's another kicker, IgG immune responses have a 26-day half-life. It takes 26 days for the body to calm down the immune response by half. So, if you have tried removing gluten for a week, you may very well have seen no relief from symptoms as the immune system is still in fighting mode weeks later. Think of this kind of immune reaction as similar to a house guest who comes to visit, stays too long and never gets the hint it is time to go. The experience is often not debilitating but can leave you tired and feeling bad.

Some people can tolerate a large amount of food without ever experiencing any outward symptoms. Others may only require a small amount of food before symptoms are expressed. The degree and severity of symptoms vary depending on the genetic makeup of the individual. Just because there is no outward sign of reaction does not mean that your immune system is not being active; it just means that your symptoms are silent or subclinical.

Clinical studies have recently been published that demonstrate how complete elimination of IgG positive foods may bring about important improvements in symptoms of IgG-mediated immune responses:

- Asthma, chronic rhinitis or sinusitis
- Chronic fatigue
- Digestive: stomach ache, irritable bowel syndrome, Crohn's Disease, ulcerative colitis and diverticulitis
- Depression and anxiety
- Headache and migraine
- Hypoglycemia
- Joint and muscle: ranging from atypical pains to rheumatoid arthritis
- Premenstrual syndrome
- Skin: itching, eczema, hives and acne (in adults)
- Sleeping disorders

While on The Cleanse Program, you will be removing the top foods that produce an IgG-delayed onsite response. In the treatment of inhalant allergies (such as asthma and hay fever) as well as food allergies (IgE) and food sensitivities (IgG), avoidance (elimination) of allergens plays an extremely important role. Now, on The Cleanse Program, you may identify some foods that are causing IgG-mediated symptoms. In this book, you will learn how to determine if you are having a reaction.

If you think you may have IgG related sensitivities, you can choose to get tested. In the case of food sensitivities, an IgG(4) food allergy panel test can help determine reactions to specific foods. This is a very different test than the standard RAST test in which the skin is pricked with the offending substance to determine if a skin-based reaction occurs. Using the blood test, an elimination/rotation diet can be specifically tailored to your personalized results.

IGA-MEDIATED IMMUNE RESPONSE: SENSITIVITY

The mucosal lining of the intestines, nose, throat and lungs are the first lines of defense against invasion and colonization by pathogenic microorganisms. In essence, mucosal surfaces in the body are the bouncer at the door with the clipboard turning away the uncool and only letting the "beautiful people" across the line.

The head honcho molecule of mucosal immune responses is Secretory IgA (SIgA). The SIgA bouncer is produced by activated immune system B-cells. Upon activation, B-cells in the mucosa form immune complexes or massive crowds (think about screaming fans trying to get an autograph from Brad Pitt in the night club—the crowd itself becomes one big mass) with the pathogens (screaming female fans) and antigens (Brad Pitt trying to get through the crowd), the ensuing melee prevents antigens (Brad Pitt) from accessing or getting through the intestinal wall (the back door). SIgA is the only immunoglobulin that can be selectively passed across mucosal walls; so it can sneak across the wall of the gut and lungs and into the blood stream.

An imbalance of protective SIgA can result in a compromised mucosal immunity and eventual gastrointestinal, immunological or neurological disorders. A deficiency of SIgA may be an indication of chronic stress, adrenal insufficiencies, bacterial colonization, a candida infection, intestinal barrier dysfunction, nutritional deficiencies, recurrent infection, autoimmune diseases such as Celiac, Crohn's, Lupus, Rheumatoid arthritis or Ulcerative Colitis.

People with low levels of SIgA are at greater risk of gastrointestinal infections, bacterial overgrowth and autoimmune disorders. Such a person may have increased IgG responses to multiple foods, or may be asymptomatic—not have any immediately identifiable symptoms to the foods causing the IgA response.

IgA-mediated responses to food and IgG-mediated responses to foods often go hand-in-hand. All of these types of immune responses have reliable and accurate testing to determine what imbalance is occurring in your gut. For more information about testing visit www.livingwelldallas.com.

The most common immune responses to foods are IgG, IgA and the extreme IgE. During The Cleanse Program, you will be removing the foods that are most common allergens in order to determine if any of your negative symptoms may be derived from dietary inputs.

4
We are What We Eat

> *Non-violence leads to the highest ethics, which is the goal of all evolution. Until we stop harming all other living beings, we are still savages.*
> *- Thomas A. Edison*

TAMMY GORA, TESTIMONIAL

I did The Cleanse Program in order to segue into a new, healthier lifestyle. At first I was scared that I would not be able to go through with it, but I quickly began to experience the effects of a healthier diet and that motivated me to stay the course.

I experienced a few caffeine withdrawal symptoms at first, but those went away within the first week. After the first week, I began seeing changes in my skin, and experienced a deeper, more restful sleep. I had no idea that food could affect my sleep patterns so much. I had struggled with sleeplessness for years. Another unexpected benefit was that I no longer experienced severe premenstrual headaches—wow!

Although losing weight was not my primary goal in participating in The Cleanse Program, I did lose weight. And even better, I lost weight in all the right areas—belly, butt, hips and thighs.

I found that there were several foods I really enjoyed that actually did not make me feel well such as wheat and dairy, but I have found other foods to replace these items in my diet.

After participating in The Cleanse Program, I have made some really positive changes to my lifestyle and now feel much better overall. I still enjoy some of the terrific recipes provided in The Cleanse Program. I have become a cheerleader for healthier eating amongst my peers at work. I am so happy with the changes my new lifestyle has had on life.

What's for supper? Never before in the history of the world has that question incited so much stress, anxiety and ultimately illness. In a country of overwhelming agricultural abundance, the quest for identifying wholesome and whole foods has become surprisingly challenging. Walk into any supermarket and you find yourself bombarded with information that is as confusing as it is misleading. Agriculture has become big business. In a consumer market where human consumption stipulates stock market success, the conventional food industry is forced to get creative in terms of how to grow their shares in an intensely competitive market.

THE PROTEIN PROBLEM

Commercial food preparations and American feedlots are perhaps the biggest change that has happened to our food supply in the last fifty years. Only fifty years ago a significant portion of the population were farmers. As a matter of fact, approximately 60 percent of Americans lived on farms. Today, less than 10 percent of Americans live on farms.

About 50 years ago, most of the animals that were raised for food were actually grass-fed and lived out their complete life in a pasture. They lived as they should—grazing on wild grasses in green pastures. For many reasons, most of them political and financial, agriculture experienced a shift to agribusiness resulting in the birth and rapid spread of the Confined Animal Feeding Operation (CAFO) where animals are kept alive standing shoulder to shoulder in incredibly unsanitary and confined spaces. Because of the massive overcrowding of the CAFO, the animals stand and live in not only their own excrement but also in the excrement of millions of other animals. To make an already unsanitary and unhealthy situation even worse, they are not fed their natural diet of grass, but rather corn. Why corn? Again, the answer is complicated and political. What is important to understand is that cows are not physiologically capable of digesting corn, and so it rots in their digestive track. The diet and the living conditions would be fatal to all of the cattle, and it is indeed fatal to many, without frequent injections of antibiotics, as well as injections of growth hormones.

So, you may be thinking, I will just eat chicken. Unfortunately, the plight of the chicken is no better. Chickens are also fed a diet of corn, which is again, not their natural diet. They live in their own CAFO as well. Chickens are packed in cages so tightly that they are literally pressed on top of one another. To prevent them from pecking and clawing one another to death, their beaks and feet are clipped (without anesthetics). Again, they would never be able to survive the terribly inhumane conditions without being pumped full of antibiotics.

Even if you are not concerned with the life these animals are living, you should be concerned about the stress they are enduring. The intense trauma they experience each day of their lives elicits the same stress hormones that would be elicited in your own body. That, and the antibiotics that are pumped into their bodies, ultimately reside in their muscle and fatty tissue, which is what becomes food. We will take a more detailed look into the meat industry and life on a CAFO in chapter five, *A Peek in the Pantry*.

THE GENETICALLY MODIFIED MESS

And if you thought it could not get worse, think again. In the last 15 to 20 years, the agricultural industry has shifted to genetically modifying the food intended for human and animal consumption. This process is also known as making it "RoundUp® Ready."

Genetically modified food originated as the brainchild of a company called Monsanto. Monsanto genetically modifies its seeds to prevent the seeds from re-seeding, and thereby forcing farmers to always purchase new seeds. The seeds must also be modified in order to meet the demands of the chemical weed killer, Roundup. Obviously, the plant needs to be able to withstand the chemical so as not to kill the food along with the weed. By altering the seed, the human body no longer responds to the genetically modified plant in the same way it responds to its natural counterpart.

The process involves inserting a DNA fragment into the DNA of the seed. It is sloppy, unpredictable and imprecise. With presently used techniques, it is impossible to guide the insertion of a gene. Therefore, it will occur haphazardly in the midst of the perfectly ordered sequence of the food's DNA.

The process includes a so-called "promoter gene" in the gene insertion packages. This promoter gene may cause metabolic disturbances. The promoter is added because it is an absolute requirement to ensure the inserted gene is "read" (i.e., copied) into RNA and translated into the protein for which it codes.

Additionally, other regulatory DNA strands called enhancers are often included as they strongly stimulate the affected gene expression. These enhancers stimulate the activity of surrounding native genes with potentially deleterious consequences. The enhancers may also activate genes that should normally be inactive. For example a toxic protein that normally is only expressed in the leaves of a food plant may become active in the fruit or seeds used.

Genetic engineering means, in most cases, the insertion of a gene coding for a protein foreign to the species. There is no way of knowing what the presence of a foreign protein will have on the metabolism and functioning of an organism, a seed or a plant.

Why should you care? Our physical health mirrors our environmental health. The illness that the human race is experiencing on a global level is a direct reflection of the illness our environment is experiencing globally. Cancer, heart disease and diabetes have all increased in the last 30 years. Obesity has increased ten-fold. What has created this shift in our national health? The only thing that we can really point to is our food supply. Exercise is not the culprit. In the early 1900s, 80 percent of the population don't exercise. Today, the number of exercisers hasn't changed. However, obesity was unheard of in 1900.

This radical shift has to do with our food and environment. Our environment is terribly toxic and not conducive to health. Our bodies were not designed to decompose industrial, foreign substances. Our bodies are not designed to ingest foods genetically modified to contain DNA from other species. By participating in the conventional food system, we are placing intense stress on our bodies, our organs and bodily processes.

So what kind of foods are the culprits in the Standard American Diet (aka: SAD diet)? The American diet has turned to fast, convenient foods that have no nutrients left in them. If you buy conventional foods and processed foods (cereals, frozen meals, TV dinners, fast food, restaurant foods, etc.) you are eating meat derived from feedlot animals and produce and grains that are most likely genetically modified. Buyer beware! Therefore, while on The Cleanse Program, it is imperative to remove these foods from the diet.

EXCITOTOXINS: TOXIC FLAVOR ENHANCERS

Excitotoxins are a class of food additives such as MSG, TVP and Aspartame that are used in fast foods, packaged foods and restaurant foods to increase the savory flavors, and increase one's desire to eat more. It is what makes soups taste more flavorful or gravies more intensely flavored. Many experts believe that excitotoxins are addictive and may be a contributor to the western obesity epidemic because they stimulate the appetite.

Excitotoxins over-activate the nervous system. Excitotoxins are compounds that attach to nerve cell receptors in the neurons. When excitotoxins are introduced, the cells rapidly and repeatedly fire nerve impulses until they reach exhaustion causing the cells to become damaged or even destroyed. The cells are literally excited to death. These chemicals also cause such widespread damage in the brain that lesions can develop. These lesions can eventually lead to Parkinson's, Amyotrophic Lateral Sclerosis (ALS), Huntington's disease and Alzheimer's disease.

In children, these excitotoxins have been implicated in developmental, learning and behavioral difficulties. Even more worrisome, when these chemicals are ingested during pregnancy, or as additives to baby and children's foods, they can increase the likelihood of endocrine disruption, hypertension, diabetes and heart disease later in life.

Excitatory neurotransmitters that occur naturally in the human body are balanced by inhibitory neurotransmitters that also naturally occur in the body. Glutamate is an excitatory neurotransmitter and amino acid that is found in abundance in the brain and is responsible for exciting the neurons. Glutamate, in its natural state in the brain, is responsible for hypothalamic endocrine function, memory and motor skills. It is considered by experts to be kept in a narrow range to manage brain neuron levels. However, ingesting large amounts of glutamate through food additives upsets this balance and causes damage to the brain cells.

The first excitotoxin on the market was Monosodium Glutamate (MSG) isolated from Kombu seaweed. Kombu seaweed is a natural sea vegetable that has been used in Japan for centuries. The Anjinomoto Company found a way to synthesize this compound by boiling vegetables in a caustic acid, neutralizing the acid with caustic soda and then drying it into a brown powder. This brown powder contains three highly dangerous toxins: glutamate, aspartate and cystoic acid.

Everyone knows that MSG is dangerous. No one would expressly choose to add it to food. So why is it still in our foods? The food industry is brilliant at the "slight of hand"—using new words to mask the ingredients consumers may be seeking to avoid. MSG is still a compound utilized in food flavoring under other less descriptive names: texturized vegetable proteins or natural flavorings, or spices. You can even find it masquerading in the bulk section of health food stores.

MSG is not the only dangerous excitotoxin over-utilized in our food supply. Aspartate, the amino acid that can damage the brain and nervous system, comprises at least 40 percent of Aspartame, the popular non-calorie sweetener NutraSweet®. When used in diet sodas, aspartate is delivered in an even more dangerous medium—its liquid form. Excitotoxins are even more damaging in liquid forms.

The one industry that has benefited most from these dangerous additives is the food manufacturing industry—fast foods, packaged foods and especially diet foods that are often void of flavor without these powerful additives.

The typical American consumes on average of 10–20 grams of the highly toxic substances per day. In laboratory studies, scientists found that humans are five times more sensitive to excitotoxins than mice. Once again, you may be wondering how these additives find their way into our foods. What about the governmental watchdog, the United States Food and Drug Administration (FDA)? Isn't the FDA charged with protecting our health?

My mom always said, "Follow the money, and you will have your answer." The food manufacturing companies and lobbying groups (including The Glutamate Association, a lobby group made up of excitotoxin manufacturers) have powerful financial ties to our economy. Their economic clout, public relation firms and spin doctors make sure that their products are seen in the most positive light in order to improve the financial gains of stock holders. The almighty dollar takes precedence over the consumers' health.

In nutrition science, you can always find two equally compelling studies with the exact opposite findings. Both studies appear to be right. In excitotoxin research, you can bet that there are studies proving the dangers. Likewise, you can find studies that prove their safety. So, how do you know whom to trust? Follow the money! Look for how the study was funded. Industry funded studies are the most questionable. What industry would harm their own financial future by publishing studies that may indicate their product is less than healthy or dangerous? Not one that is the fifth largest industry in the world and dependent on the substance being studied.

Do you really want these additives in your body? What about your children's body?

Ingredient Additive Names that contain Excitotoxins:

- Aspartame
- Aspartate
- Autolyzed protein
- Bouillon
- Calcium caseinate
- Cysteine or cystoic Acid
- Hydrolyzed protein
- Hydrolyzed vegetable protein
- Malt extract
- Malt flavoring
- MSG
- Monosodium glutamate
- Natural beef or chicken flavors
- Natural flavoring seasonings
- Plant protein extract
- Spices
- Stock flavoring
- Yeast extract

GLUTEN SENSITIVITY

Celiac disease is the most common genetic disease. Although an estimated one in 4,700 Americans have been diagnosed with this disease, according to the Celiac Disease Foundation as many as one in every 133 people may have it and over 97% go undiagnosed. The Gluten Intolerance Group postulates that 1 in every 110 people in the U.S. may have celiac disease, which is only one presentation of gluten related autoimmunity with untold others suffering a muriad of conditions in which gluten has been shown to play a roll.

What is Gluten?

Gluten is a cohesive, elastic protein found in wheat, rye, spelt and barley. It gives bread its characteristic creamy and fluffy texture. Gluten is made up of proteins classified in two groups, the polyamines and the glutelins.

Gliadin is a prolamine and it seems to be the catalyst in Celiac disease. For a gluten intolerant person, this offending substance causes inflammation including damaging the lining of the small intestines flattening the small finger-like projections or villi that normally protrude from the intestinal surfaces to absorb nutrients from food.

What is Celiac Disease?

Joseph Murray, MD of Baystr University defines Celiac disease as a permanent intolerance to gluten that results in damage to the small intestine and is reversible with avoidance of dietary gluten and gluten-containing grains.

Because the villi become damaged, they are unable to absorb water and nutrients making the Celiac sufferer susceptible to a variety of other conditions related to mal-absorption such as anemia or osteoporosis. But, you do not have to be a full-blown Celiac to experience problems with gluten sensitivities.

There are several conditions that fall into the gluten-sensitivity continuum. At one end are wheat allergies. These are simple IgE-mediated allergies. You may remember that IgE-mediated allergies are the classic type of allergies which result in obvious immediate symptoms such as hives, breathing difficulty and asphyxia. IgE allergies are easy to test for and definitively diagnose.

Then there is what is referred to as "gluten sensitivity" or "gluten intolerance." Some people may actually have Celiac disease or dermatitis herpetiformis, but because their testing methods were not specific for Celiac disease or because their health care practitioner did not know to look for Celiac disease, they were told they have a gluten sensitivity or intolerance. Some people who fall in this category do not test positive for Celiac disease but are considered "sub-clinical," meaning it is likely that they would test positive in the future if they were to continue to eat gluten. Others may simply be sensitive to gluten and still test negative. These people often feel better when they avoid gluten-containing foods.

At the other end of the spectrum is Celiac disease or dermatitis herpetiformis (DH). Celiac disease is a genetic autoimmune condition. People with Celiac disease must strictly comply with a gluten-free diet because the immune response damages the small intestine. Celiac disease is a serious disease.

Symptoms

The symptoms of Celiac disease can vary with each individual. They can range from no symptoms at all to severe gas, bloating, diarrhea and abdominal pain as well as neurological changes such as seizures, migraines, mood swings and even schizophrenia. In its most aggressive form, if untreated, malnutrition can occur. If left untreated too long, celiac disease can be life-threatening. Yes, symptoms do not always involve the digestive system. Celiac can cause irritability, depression, muscle cramps, joint pain, fatigue, menstrual irregularities and mineral absorption problems just to name a few.

Diagnosis

Blood antibody tests (endomysial, reticulin (IgA), tissue transglutaminase and gliadin (IgG and IgA) are easy to use to measure levels of antibodies to gluten and can be an indicator of damage. If the antibodies in the blood are higher than normal then a biopsy of the small intestine is done. A biopsy of the lining of the small intestine checks for damage to the villi. If the villi appear damaged then a gluten-free diet is introduced. Another biopsy is done after six months or more of dieting. Relief of symptoms or reversal of an abnormal intestinal biopsy is the most convincing evidence that an individual has Celiac disease or gluten sensitivity.

Beware! The Celiac community is littered with people who have had false negative biopsies. These people may go years before obtaining an accurate biopsy all the while consuming gluten. Because the small intestines are large enough to fill a tennis court with folds and crevices as well as finger-like projections, damage to intestines from Celiac disease does not occur in a uniform manner. A biopsy can very easily be taken from an area of the intestine that has not yet been damaged. The blood tests, if positive, are all you need to know to remove gluten from your diet.

Who is at Risk?

Celiac disease is hereditary and was thought to primarily affect Caucasians of northwestern European, Irish and English ancestry. Celiac is less likely to affect people of African and Jewish descent, people of Asian descent and people of Mediterranean ancestry. Ancestries aside, people of all different races have been diagnosed with Celiac disease and Gluten Intolerance. If you have the symptoms listed above, the simple blood tests for the genes associated with gluten sensitivity and anti-gliadin antibodies may be the best money you will ever spend to improve your health.

But isn't Celiac disease a childhood disease? According to a recent study by Department of Medicine, Harbor-UCLA Medical Center in Torrance, California, Celiac disease is more often found in adults than children. The largest population of a nationwide patient support group for Celiac disease was surveyed to determine their onset of severe symptoms and time of diagnosis. In the initial survey of 1032 respondents, the median age at symptom onset was 46 years, and the diagnosis of adult celiac disease was often delayed. The median delay was 12 months with 21% delayed over 10 years. Of those respondents, only 32% of adults were underweight, and only about 50% reported frequent diarrhea and weight loss. Initial physician diagnoses were often irritable bowel syndrome (37%), psychological disorders (29%), and fibromyalgia (9%).

So Celiac disease is not just a childhood disease. Many people are silent only to have symptoms appear after severe stress, emotional or physical trauma, surgery or a viral infection. Symptoms may slowly appear over time with increasing levels of severity. And a significant number of diagnosed Celiacs never present with outward symptoms.

It is important to note that a person can be allergic to another protein in wheat and not allergic or sensitive to the gluten or gliadin protein. Some people with wheat allergies are not gluten/gliadin intolerant or Celiac and can eat rye, barley and spelt. These individuals must only remove wheat from their diet.

Treatment

The only acceptable treatment for Celiac disease or Gluten Intolerance requires a life-time adherence to a strict avoidance of all products that contain gluten. An adherence to a gluten-free diet can prevent almost all complications caused by the disease. Reading product food labels is vital. Wheat is not the only offender; watch out for other offending grains such as rye, oats and barley. Remember products labeled wheat-free are not necessarily gluten-free. Gluten is in many forms of processed foods and has a lot of names it hides under.

Avoid foods with the following ingredients:

- Caramel color: This additive results from a controlled heat treatment of dextrose (corn sugar), invert sugar, lactose (milk sugar), malt syrup (usually from barley malt), molasses (from cane), starch hydrolysis (can include wheat) or sucrose (cane or beet).
- Cereal: cereal grains and cereal flour unless labeled gluten-free
- Colorings and dyes artificial flavors: Often the source of the dye is not on the label. Some people report allergic reactions.
- Undistilled vinegar: flavored vinegars and malt vinegars
- Emulsifiers: Emulsifiers alter the surface properties of other ingredients they contact; emulsifiers may contain gluten from grain.
- Enriched flour or flour
- Gluten peptides: Gluten peptides are smaller pieces of protein from wheat, barley, rye, oats and other grains. These certain peptides produce intestinal damage in Celiacs.
- Hydrolyzed Vegetable Protein: Hydrolyzed plant protein and Textured

Vegetable Protein - HVP, HPP and TVP usually are made from wheat, corn or soy.

- Lectins/Lecithins: May be from the hull or grain coat of soy, amaranth, barley or other grains.
- Malt: Malt is usually made from barley. May be made from corn.
- Malto-Dextrose: Maltose and dextrins that may be obtained by enzymatic action of barley malt or acorn flour. Celiacs must avoid this product if the source is unknown.
- Modified food starch or starch: U.S. manufacturers' ingredient "starch" is cornstarch only (not true for foreign manufactures or pharmaceuticals). "Modified food starch" may be made from wheat, corn, arrowroot, potato, tapioca or maize.
- Monosodium glutamate: Foreign sources of MSG usually contain gluten-containing grains.
- Natural flavor: By definition, natural flavor may or may not contain any of the gluten-containing grains or derivatives.
- Semolina or durum
- Triticale: Triticale is a new grain that was created by crossing rye and durum wheat. Its kernels are longer than wheat seeds and are plumper than rye.

Gluten is often used as a thickener. Be sure to read the labels on canned soups, catsups, mustards, soy sauce and other condiments (many contain gluten). The only way to know for sure that gluten is not in the processed food is to buy foods that are labeled gluten-free. Treatment, or in this case, a gluten-free diet, is important because people with Celiac disease could develop complications such as cancer, osteoporosis, anemia, infertility and seizures.

Related Disorders

Celiac disease is linked to many immune related disorders. The best-established connection is with Type I diabetes (mellitus). Gluten sensitivity has been implicated in osteoporosis, fertility problems, obesity, vitamin and mineral deficiencies and as a factor in mood disorders, ADD and ADHD. Many people suffer from these kinds of health issues related to gluten intolerance and do not know it because they do not suffer the "traditional" digestive maladies associated with food sensitivities. If you eat gluten-containing grains and are sensitive, you may experience no obvious ill-side effects.

Some other illnesses related to Celiac disease are chronic, active hepatitis, chronic fatigue syndrome and inflammatory bowel disease. Some researchers believe that gluten intolerance can impair mental functioning in some individuals. They also believe it can cause or aggravate autism, attention deficit disorder (ADD) and schizophrenia. Since gluten can damage the villi, it is also common for Celiacs to have problems with other food sensitivities due to leaky gut and an inability to digest dairy. Damage to the gut creates an environment where malnutrition may occur through poor absorption of nutrients.

SUGAR

How bad is sugar, *really*? Did you know that the body maintains an average of one to one-and-a-half teaspoon of sugar in the form of glucose circulating in your blood stream? Any amounts over that will require insulin to either store it as fat or shuttle the glucose across the cell walls for energy production. So, think about this: the average soda pop or canned fruit juice can contain 12–17 teaspoons of sugar or more. Imagine what the consumption of these common foods does to our insulin management system.

The white crystalline substance we know as sugar is an unnatural substance produced by industrial processes derived mostly from sugar cane or sugar beets. The process removes all vital nutrients from the previously healthy foods by refining it down to pure sucrose—stripping away all the vitamins, minerals, proteins, enzymes and other beneficial nutrients. What is left is a concentrated unnatural substance the human body is not able to effectively detoxify, especially in the quantities that are ingested in today's Standard American Diet.

Sugar is addictive and utilizes the same receptor sites in the brain as opiates. In the early 1900s, the average consumption of sugar was only five pounds per person per year. The average American now consumes approximately 150 pounds or more of sugar per year. This is per man, woman and child.

The body cannot utilize this refined starch and carbohydrate (Read: the white stuff) unless the depleted proteins, vitamins and minerals are present. Remember, the word vitamin came from the "vital amine" - necessary for life. Yes, vitamins, minerals and amino acids are required for your body's metabolism to function and break down foods. Nature supplies these elements in each plant in quantities sufficient to metabolize the carbohydrate in that particular plant.

Incomplete carbohydrate metabolism results in the formation of toxic metabolite such as pyruvic acid. Pyruvic acid accumulates in the brain and nervous system and the abnormal sugars in the red blood cells. These toxic metabolites interfere with the respiration or breathing of the cells. Cellular respiration is the process of oxidizing or breaking down of food molecules, such as glucose, to carbon dioxide and water. The energy released through this process is trapped in the form of Adenosine 5'-triphosphate (ATP) for use by all the energy-consuming activities of the cell. If the cells cannot get sufficient oxygen to survive and function normally, in time, some of the cells die.

Even more concerning, fructose, high fructose corn syrup and corn sugar, especially the highly refined stuff you find in every thing; metabolize differently in the body and cause rapid damage of the mitochondria (powerhouse of the cell)and a depletion of ATP leading to energy loss and sugars in the diet to be stored as fat. According to Dr. Lyn Patrick fructose amounts over 50g a day will create fatty liver that can progress toward liver damage and cirrhosis, weight gain and insulin resistance. Fructose that is not in its natural form in fruits should be removed from your diet and the total sugar intake for one day should be less than 45g a day if you are trying to lose weight or are concerned about any of the conditions on pages 60 and 61.

Sugar taken every day produces a continuously over-acidic condition in the blood stream, and more and more minerals are required from the body in the attempt to rectify the imbalance and reduce the acidity. Sugar leaches the body of precious vitamins and minerals through the demand it makes on digestion, detoxification and elimination. Minerals such as sodium (from salt), potassium and magnesium (from vegetables), and calcium (from the bones) are mobilized and used in an attempt to return the acid-alkaline balance of the blood to normal levels.

Excess sugar eventually affects every organ in the body. Initially, it is stored in the liver in the form of glucose (glycogen). When the liver is filled to its maximum capacity, the excess glycogen is returned to the blood in the form of fatty acids (Read: plain old FAT). These are taken to every part of the body and stored in the most inactive areas— the belly, the buttocks, the breasts and thighs.

When these comparatively harmless places are completely filled, fatty acids are then distributed among active organs, such as the heart and kidneys. These organs begin to slow down, and eventually their tissues degenerate and turn to fat. The whole body is affected by their reduced ability, and abnormal blood pressure is created. The parasympathetic nervous system is affected. The circulatory and lymphatic systems are invaded. The immune system is compromised and is less likely to be able to fight potential invading organisms. The whole body is degraded and clogged with fat.

Sugar: A Game of Hide & Seek

Sugar is often well hidden in sneaky labeling techniques used by the processed foods industry. Look at any food label, and you will see the carbohydrate count listed. The use of the word "carbohydrate" to describe sugar is intentionally misleading.

Since the 1994 Nutrition Labeling and Education Act (NLEA), improvements have been made in the labeling of nutritional properties on packages and cans. However, there are sneaky "loopholes" that allow refined carbohydrates such as sugar to be lumped together with other carbohydrates that may or may not be refined. Several types of carbohydrates are added together for an overall carbohydrate total. Thus, the effect of the label is to hide the sugar content from the unsuspecting buyer. To add to the confusion, food chemists use the word "sugar" to describe an entire group of sugar substances that are similar but not identical.

Sugar in processed foods could be any combination of the following:

- Glucose: A sugar found usually with other sugars, such as fructose in fruits and vegetables. Glucose is often called "blood sugar."
- Dextrose: Also called "corn sugar," dextrose is derived synthetically from cornstarch.
- Fructose: A fruit sugar. But can also be seen as fructose corn syrup or high fructose corn syrup or now labeled as "corn sugar".
- Maltose: A malt sugar usually created from grains such as barley.
- Lactose: A milk sugar.
- Sucrose: A refined sugar made from sugar cane and sugar beet.

The body metabolizes each of these sugars differently. For example: Scientists now are finding that fructose corn syrup is a leading contributor to inflammation and elevated triglycerides and is much more detrimental to one's health than sucrose. Any combination of these types of sugars can be labeled as just sugar. Consumers must look at the ingredients to understand the whole picture.

What Exactly is Sugar?

Sugar of all kinds, including natural sugars such as those in honey and fruit (fructose) as well as the refined white stuff (sucrose), tends to slow the secretion of gastric juices and has an inhibiting effect on peristalsis (movement) of the stomach. Unlike animal proteins, sugars are quickly assimilated. When eaten alone, they pass quickly through the stomach into the small intestine and into the blood stream unencumbered. When sugars are eaten with other foods, especially fiber, fat or protein, they are held up in the stomach for a while and released more slowly to the small intestines.

Enzymes enable the breakdown of foods into their small nutrient parts to be used in functions and repair. Fermentation or bacterial decomposition creates toxins. When starches and sugars are eaten together and undergo fermentation, the sugars are broken down into carbon dioxide, acetic acid, alcohol and water. With the exception of the water, all of these are unusable substances that must be detoxified by the body. When proteins are eaten with significant amounts of sugar, they putrefy and are broken into a variety of substances including ptomaine—an alkaloid produced by bacteria that is responsible for body decomposition.

William Dufty provides a list of the effects of sugar on the body in his book, *Sugar Blues* (available on Amazon.com and at most health foods stores). A partial and paraphrased list is available below:

- Sugar can suppress your immune system and impair your defenses against infectious disease.

- Sugar upsets the mineral relationships in your body causing chromium and copper deficiencies and interferes with absorption of calcium and magnesium.

- Sugar can cause a rapid rise of adrenaline, hyperactivity, anxiety, difficulty concentrating and crankiness in children.

- Sugar can produce a significant rise in total cholesterol, triglycerides and bad cholesterol and a decrease in good cholesterol.

- Sugar causes a loss of tissue elasticity and function.

- Sugar feeds cancer cells and has been connected with the development of cancer of the breast, ovaries, prostate, rectum, pancreas, biliary tract, lung, gallbladder and stomach.

- Sugar can increase fasting levels of glucose causing reactive hypoglycemia.

- Sugar can weaken eyesight.
- Sugar can cause many problems with the gastrointestinal tract including the following: an acidic digestive tract, indigestion, mal-absorption in patients with functional bowel disease, increased risk of Crohn's disease and ulcerative colitis.
- Sugar can cause premature aging.
- Sugar can lead to alcoholism.
- Sugar can cause your saliva to become acidic leading to tooth decay and periodontal disease.
- Sugar contributes to obesity.
- Sugar can cause autoimmune diseases such as arthritis, asthma and multiple sclerosis.
- Sugar greatly assists the uncontrolled growth of Candida Albicans (yeast infections).
- Sugar can cause gallstones.
- Sugar can cause appendicitis.
- Sugar can cause hemorrhoids.
- Sugar can cause varicose veins.
- Sugar can elevate glucose and insulin responses in oral contraceptive users.
- Sugar can contribute to osteoporosis.
- Sugar can cause a decrease in your insulin sensitivity thereby causing an abnormally high insulin levels and eventually diabetes.
- Sugar can lower vitamin E levels.
- Sugar can increase systolic blood pressure.
- Sugar can cause drowsiness and decreased activity in children.
- High sugar intake increases advanced glycation end products (AGEs). (i.e., Sugar molecules attach to and thereby damage proteins in the body).
- Sugar can interfere with the absorption of protein.
- Sugar causes food allergies.
- Sugar can cause toxemia during pregnancy.
- Sugar can contribute to eczema in children.

- Sugar can cause atherosclerosis and cardiovascular disease.
- Sugar can impair the structure of your DNA.
- Sugar can change the structure of protein and cause a permanent alteration of the way the proteins act in your body.
- Sugar can make skin age by changing the structure of collagen.
- Sugar can cause cataracts and nearsightedness.
- Sugar can cause emphysema.
- High sugar intake can impair the physiological homeostasis of many systems in your body.
- Sugar lowers the ability of enzymes to function.
- Sugar intake is higher in people with Parkinson's disease.
- Sugar can increase the size of your liver by making your liver cells divide and it can increase the amount of liver fat.
- Sugar can increase kidney size and produce pathological changes in the kidney such as the formation of kidney stones.
- Sugar can damage pancreas.
- Sugar can increase body's fluid retention.
- Sugar can compromise the ability to have regular bowel movements.
- Sugar can compromise the lining of your capillaries.
- Sugar can make tendons more brittle.
- Sugar can cause headaches, including migraines.
- Sugar can reduce a child's capacity for learning, adversely affect school grades and cause learning disorders.
- Sugar can cause an increase in delta, alpha and theta brain waves, which can alter your mind's ability to think clearly.
- Sugar can cause depression.
- Sugar can increase the risk of gout.
- Sugar can increase the risk of Alzheimer's disease.
- Sugar can cause hormonal imbalances such as increase estrogen in men, exacerbate PMS and decrease growth hormone.

- Sugar can lead to dizziness.
- Diets high in sugar will increase free radicals and oxidative stress.
- People with peripheral vascular disease who consume a high sucrose diet have a significantly increased risk of platelet adhesion leading to an increase in blood clot formation.
- High sugar consumption in pregnant adolescents can lead to a substantial decrease in gestation duration and is associated with a twofold, increased risk for delivering a small-for-gestational-age (SGA) infant.
- Sugar is an addictive substance.
- Sugar can be intoxicating, similar to alcohol.
- When given to premature babies, sugar can affect the amount of carbon dioxide they produce.
- Decrease in sugar intake can increase emotional stability.
- Your body changes sugar into two to five times more fat in the bloodstream than it does starch.
- The rapid absorption of sugar promotes excessive food intake in obese subjects.
- Sugar can worsen the symptoms of children with attention deficit hyperactivity disorder (ADHD).
- Sugar adversely affects urinary electrolyte composition.
- Sugar can slow down the functioning of your adrenal glands.
- Sugar has the potential of inducing abnormal metabolic processes in a normal, healthy individual and promotes chronic degenerative diseases.
- Intravenous feedings of sugar water can cut off oxygen to your brain.
- Sugar increases the risk of polio.
- High sugar intake can cause epileptic seizures.
- Sugar causes high blood pressure in obese people.
- In intensive care units, limiting sugar saves lives.
- Sugar may induce cell death.
- In juvenile rehabilitation camps, when children were put on a low-sugar diet, there was a 44 percent drop in antisocial behavior.
- Sugar dehydrates newborns.

THE DAIRY DILEMMA

What do you think when you see movie actors and athletes with a white mustache on their lips? Do you think that milk really "does a body good"? Or that milk strengthens bones? There is little data to support any health benefits from drinking milk including the claims that it strengthens bones and assists in weight loss.

Beyond lactose intolerance, which is when the body's inability to produce the enzyme lactase to breakdown the lactose sugar in milk, many people are sensitive to casein, and in some cases, the whey protein in dairy. Casein and whey are the two main protein components to dairy foods.

A study from Harvard Medical School found that men who drink more than four glasses of milk per day are at higher risk for prostate cancer than those who do not. The researchers explain that calcium in milk sequesters the vitamin D in the milk itself and from the body reserves. Although the milk manufacturers add vitamin D to milk, there is not enough available in the milk to offset the loss of vitamin D caused by the body's attempt at metabolizing the calcium in milk. Statistically, regular milk drinkers have lower blood levels of vitamin D than those who do not drink milk. A lack of vitamin D causes cancer.

The data does not show that milk prevents osteoporosis. Several studies show that osteoporosis is far more associated with low levels of vitamin D, a diet high in acid producing foods, mal-absorption and consuming too much protein relative to vegetables and fruits, as opposed to not getting enough calcium in the diet. The kidneys respond to these events by neutralizing the acid by taking calcium from bones and excreting it through the urine.

Got Asthma, Allergies and Mucus?

If you suffer from a chronic runny nose and sore throat, it might be time to dump the dairy. According to the American Academy of Allergy, Asthma and Immunology, cow's milk is the number one cause of food allergies in children. According to the former director of pediatrics at Johns Hopkins University, Dr. Frank Oski, there is evidence to indicate that up to half of U.S. children experience some degree of allergy to milk. And kids grow up to be adults. For these kids and adults, milk plays a synergistic role in persistent problems such as sinus congestion, asthma and ear infections. I have seen this again and again in my clients—their sinus and asthma symptoms disappear when they stop consuming dairy, and they reappear when they eat dairy. Coincidence? I think not.

According to a study published by the American Academy of Allergy and Immunology Committee on Adverse Reactions to Food (part of the National Institutes of Health), the allergies of up to one-third of the children tested cleared after milk was removed from their diet. In her book, *Women's Body's Women's Wisdom,* Dr. Christiane Northrup asserts, "Dairy is a tremendous mucus producer and a burden on the respiratory, digestive, and immune systems."

Got Acne or Backcne?

Canadian dermatologist Dr. F.W. Danby reported in a 2005 article published in the medical journal *Dermatology* that dairy has been linked as a cause of acne. He concluded drinking milk and consuming dairy products from pregnant cows exposes us to the hormones produced by the cows' pregnancy hormones. Humans are not designed to consume cow hormones. He surmised that these hormones had an effect on the sebaceous glands in the skin that in turn clogged the pores. He found that removing dairy for a significant time in the diet caused the reaction to subside.

More Cheese Please?

Casein is a protein found in milk and foods containing milk, such as cheese, butter, yogurt, ice cream, whey and even some brands of vegetarian replacement foods such as soy cheese and veggie hot dogs in the form of caseinate.

Casein sensitivities have been implicated in a number of neurological and digestive complaints such as mood and cognitive disorders including autistic spectrum, ADD and ADHD, colitis, Crohn's disease, IBS and eczema.

The Casein/Autism Connection

There is growing interest in the link between autism and gastrointestinal (GI) ailments. According to one theory, some people with autism and other behavioral disorders cannot properly digest casein and gluten from wheat. When we break down casein, the process forms peptides into caso-morphine (that's right, morphine, as in the drug), that act like opiates (drug) docking in our opiate receptors in the brain. The caso-morphine peptides then alter the person's behavior, perceptions and responses to the environment. Some scientists now believe that peptides trigger an unusual immune system response in certain people. I have always said this is why "Cheese people are major cheese people." You know who you are. You cannot live without cheese! This opiate component might very well be what is driving that craving. I know, because I *love* cheese, but

I drastically limit its intake. Once I eat cheese, it is like a drug; I want more and more. Your experience may be similar.

Casein and Cancer

In his book, *The China Study*, Dr. T. Colin Campbell discovered, over many years of cancer research, a possible link between animal protein intake and cancer development. In the early 1980s, a joint effort was established between Cornell University, Oxford University and China's health research laboratory. The researchers gathered data on 367 variables, across 65 counties in China and 6,500 adults. The research was conducted over a 10-year period and was funded by both the Chinese and the United States governments.

He found that protein did indeed promote cancer development. However it was not all types of protein. Casein, which comprises 85 percent of the protein in cow's milk, promoted cancer in all stages of its development. In fact, the connection between casein and cancer was so profound that the scientists could literally turn cancer growth on and off in the laboratory animals, like a light switch, simply by altering the level of casein protein in their diets. Interestingly, they also found that feeding the animals the same levels of plant-based protein did not at all promote cancer growth.

On The Cleanse Program, you will not be consuming dairy products. This will enable you to experience the effects it has in your body. After the cleanse, you can consume dairy if you like, but you should not think that it has any special health benefits.

SOY THE "HEALTH FOOD OF THE CENTURY"

Over the past 15 years, soy foods have become America's favorite health food. Magazines, marketers and manufacturers have proclaimed the "joy of soy" and promoted the belief that soy food is the key to disease prevention and maximum longevity. Americans rarely hear anything negative about soy. Thanks to the strong and financially fortified soy interests. Wow, wouldn't it be nice if an inexpensive plant food could really prevent heart disease, fight cancer, halt hot flashes and build strong bones? The truth, unfortunately, is far more complex. Soy comes in a variety of forms and is included in almost all processed foods.

Soy has been touted as a health food and especially marketed for women. However, new studies question whether the ingredients in soy might increase the risk of breast cancer in some women, affect brain function in men and lead to hidden developmental abnormalities in infants. The core concerns are the chemical makeup of soy, specifically the natural chemical, phytoestrogens that mimics estrogen, the female sex hormone. Some studies in animals show that this chemical can alter sexual hormone function. In fact, two glasses of soymilk per day, over the course of one month, contains enough of the chemical to change the timing of a woman's menstrual cycle.

Soybeans also contain isoflavones. Isoflavones are the compounds that are being studied to determine if they may play a role in relieving certain menopausal symptoms, reducing cancer risk, slowing or reversing bone loss and reducing the risk of heart disease.

Soybeans, as found in nature, are not suitable for human consumption. Only after considerable fermentation, or extensive processing, are the beans or the sub-fractions of nutrients from soy suitable for digestion when eaten. Even natural forms of soy foods should be eaten sparingly, as they have been for years in Asia.

But don't Asians eat large quantities of soy every day and consequently remain free of most western diseases? Not really. In fact, the people of Asia eat very little soy other than soy sauce, natto, tempeh and tofu. These soy foods are eaten sparingly, not three times a day as significant portions of a meal. And they are fermented which alters the nutritional components of soy considerably.

For years, the soy protein left over from soybean oil processing went to animal feed, not human foods. Now that food scientists have discovered inexpensive ways to disguise the color and flavor of soy protein-based products, soy is being aggressively marketed as a super health food.

Soy contains components that are not friendly to the human body. Here are just a few:

- Oligosaccharides give soy and other beans its notorious reputation as a gas producer.
- Soy contains protease inhibitors, which interfere with protein digestion and have caused malnutrition, poor growth and digestive issues.
- Oxalates in soy may cause problems for people prone to kidney stones. Oxalates also have been shown to contribute to vulvodynia, a painful condition marked by burning, stinging and itching of the external genitalia.
- Phytates in soy and other beans block mineral absorption causing mineral deficiencies.

- Lectins and saponins have caused leaky gut and other gastrointestinal and immune problems.

Soy is one of the top eight allergens that cause IgE-mediated (immediate hypersensitivity) reactions such as coughing, sneezing, runny nose, hives, diarrhea, difficulty swallowing and anaphylactic shock. IgG-mediated or delayed allergic responses are even more common and have been linked to sleep disturbances, joint paint, chronic fatigue and gastrointestinal woes.

Soy allergies are on the rise from the increase in soy-containing foods in grocery stores and the possibility of the greater allergenicity of genetically modified soybeans. If you do not believe you are eating a lot of soy, just turn over your box of processed foods and read the label. It is cheap, abundant and has an infinite number of ways it can be used to mimic other foods.

The bottom line is that the safety of eating significant amounts soy foods has yet to be proven. While on The Cleanse Program you will not be eating soy so that you can determine if soy is causing a problem for you.

CONCERNS WITH CORN

Unless you work in the corn industry, or already know you are allergic to the stuff, it is hard to grasp just how much of the grocery store is made of corn. Corn chips, corn tortillas and fresh corn are the obvious culprits. But then there is cornmeal and cornstarch, corn oil and corn syrup, corn as a thickener or a sweetener or just an invisible additive.

In its whole form, corn is a cheap, filling source of starch and vitamins, and its obvious versatility has made it a culinary staple in the United States. But only the tiniest fraction of our corn supply ends up boiled and buttered or even converted to cornmeal. Given current farm bills and modern commodity agriculture, large-scale corn producers receive government subsidies—to the tune of four billion dollars a year making this crop ludicrously cheap.

The government subsidies create the incentive to sell corn in every possible form. And since we can only eat so much corn on the cob, the industry has conjured all sorts of corn-based derivatives. As a result, consumers end up with corn processed beyond recognition into forms that eliminate virtually all of its nutritional content.

Corn Syrup

Consumption of corn syrup has increased more than 1000 percent between 1970 and 1990, according to Nina Planck, author of *Real Food*. Its sudden debut, especially corn derivatives and high fructose corn syrup, into the American diet corresponds almost exactly to a dramatic climb in obesity rates.

Corn plays an omnipresent and nefarious role in a recent book, *The Omnivore's Dilemma*, in which author Michael Pollan reveals that, at the molecular level, Americans have ingested so many corn-derived substances that we are essentially walking corn chips. The post WWII boom in synthetic fertilizer (from bomb-making ammonium) enabled farmers to grow vast quantities of corn without having to rotate crops as had been done in the past. Corn pushed out pasture-raised cattle, pigs and chickens, as it became the ubiquitous agricultural crop.

The following is just a taste of the amount of corn-derived carbon Pollan found in his experiment with one McDonald's® family meal, as measured by a mass spectrometer:

- Soda: 100 percent corn
- Milkshake: 78 percent corn
- Salad dressing: 65 percent corn
- Chicken nuggets: 56 percent corn
- Cheeseburger: 52 percent corn
- French fries: 23 percent corn

In his book, *The Omnivore's Dilemma*, Pollan asserts, "Corn is in the coffee creamer and Cheez Whiz®, the frozen yogurt and TV dinner, the canned fruit and ketchup and candies, the soups and snacks and cake mixes...everything from the toothpaste and cosmetics to the disposable diapers, trash bags, cleansers, charcoal briquettes, matches, and batteries, right down to the shine of the magazine that catches your eye by the checkout: corn."

Getting Out of the Maize

"To start, it's a problem from a health point of view," claims Pollan, explaining that as omnivores, humans need about 50 different nutrients and atoms—amino acids, minerals, phytochemicals, fat, sugar, etc. "A lot of people eating a fast-food diet—not just the drive-through kind, but also microwaveable and other prepackaged meals—are malnourished."

Other bigger, hidden costs are also associated with corn-based cheap food. "We pay with our taxes, because it takes heavy, heavy government subsidies to produce food that cheaply," he says. "We pay with the public health system, with failing antibiotics (whose overuse in cattle has given rise to new antibiotic-resistant strains of 'super-bugs'). We pay with the miles-wide dead zone in the Gulf of Mexico (caused by nitrate-dense agricultural runoff carried out by the Mississippi River). We pay by having to defend our high-energy food system by fighting wars in the Middle East."

Eliminating Corn From a Diet

There are no cures for a food allergy or sensitivity other than removing the offending substance and corn is one of the top foods that appear on IgG and IgE testing results. So removing corn during a cleanse is required. However, avoiding corn is not as easy as it may initially seem. If you consume packaged, fast and prepared foods, it is not as simple as not eating corn-on-the-cob or staying away from corn syrup.

There are common symptoms one may experience if an allergy to corn is present. Allergists and other traditional medical professionals tend to only recognize the traditional symptoms; the non-traditional symptoms tend to be those family members identify.

Traditional Symptoms (IgE-Mediated)

- Anaphylaxis
- Asthma attacks and/or shortness of breath
- Breathing and/or swallowing difficulties
- Drop in blood pressure
- Intestinal issues, such as stomach discomfort/cramps/pain, diarrhea, nausea and/or vomiting
- Migraine headaches
- Rashes and/or hives
- Tongue, face and/or throat swelling and/or tingling

Non-Traditional Symptoms (IgG-Mediated)

- Depression
- Disturbed sleep

- Eczema
- Fatigue
- Fuzzy thinking
- Joint pains
- Hyperactivity (especially in children)
- Inability to concentrate
- Lethargy
- Mood swings and/or behavioral changes (especially in children)
- Night sweats
- Raccoon eyes or allergy shiners
- Recurring ear infections
- Respiratory conditions
- Sinus conditions
- Urinary tract infections (UTI)

So now that you know that corn is everywhere, do you feel like you are a kernel of corn?

ACIDIC BEANS

Beans are for most people a healthy addition to the diet. For some people, beans increase digestive discomfort such as gas and bloating. Several beans are included on The Cleanse Program with the exception of kidney beans, pinto beans and navy beans. These beans are the most acidic and increase the level of acidity of the body.

Some types of raw beans, especially red beans and kidney beans, contain the harmful toxin phytohemagglutinin. This toxin must be removed by soaking and then cooking the beans. Note: If you are cooking beans from scratch, the soaking water from beans should be discarded before boiling, and they should be boiled for at least ten minutes. In addition, beans contain high levels of lectins which can activate your immune system causing symptoms.

Many edible beans contain oligosaccharides. The oligosaccharidase enzyme is necessary to properly digest these sugar molecules. A normal human digestive tract does not contain the oligosaccharidase enzyme. Consumed oligosaccharides are typically digested not by the small intestines but rather by bacteria in the large intestine. This digestion process produces flatulence, which causes gas as a by-product. So guess what? You must have a good balance of intestinal bacteria in order to digest beans. If you get gassy, you may have a digestive tract that is out of balance.

To reduce the flatulence effects of beans, they can be cooked along with natural carminatives such as anise seeds, coriander seeds and cumin. Other strategies include soaking beans in water for several hours before mixing them with other ingredients to remove the offending sugars. Sometimes vinegar is added, but only after the beans are cooked as vinegar interferes with the beans' softening.

HIGH SUGAR FRUIT AND SELECTED CITRUS

Many of the tropical fruits such as pineapple, orange, tangerines, banana and mangos also contain higher levels of fructose, the sugar found mostly in fruits. For The Cleanse Program, you will be reducing the amount of sugar circulating and putting stress on the pancreas and insulin production. These fruits will be off the cleanse.

Also, fructose sugar has been known to cause digestive distress. Some folks have trouble digesting the pulp, leading to rather spectacular diarrhea. Fructose has also been implicated in increasing uric acid and insulin resistance. Many of the citric foods can also wreak havoc on people with acid reflux, ulcers or other sourness sensitivities. They also cause problems for people with Crohn's, IBD and IBS. Citric fruits can cause rashes on the skin or a rash around lips.

For those people who may be struggling with digestive disorders such as GERD, ulcerative colitis or Crohn's, you may have already found that the citrus family of foods causes an exacerbation of symptoms. You may want to exclude even the allowed citrus of lemon, lime and grapefruit on The Cleanse Program.

COFFEE AND YOUR CAFFEINE FIX

If the FDA had to approve caffeine as a food additive today, they would decline approval. When extracted from foods, caffeine becomes a white powder that causes many adverse affects when consumed. Now, you might wonder why it is so prevalent in our society. Caffeine containing foods, especially coffee, are ubiquitous in our collective culture; so it has been effectively grandfathered in as a safe component of foods.

We all like a good cup of coffee once in a while (some more frequently than others). And a good cup of organic coffee on a cold day can be a great source of physical, mental and even emotional comfort. But caffeine, and particularly coffee, can cause digestive discomfort. During your cleanse, you will be weaning yourself from your coffee addiction. Not sure if you are a coffee addict? Try skipping a day or two of your morning coffee. If you get a slamming headache and feel rundown, congratulations you are addicted! This can be fixed in a short time. If you can skip a few days between hits, then you are not addicted.

Effects of Coffee on the Body

A study conducted by researchers at Duke University Medical Center funded by the National Institutes of Health, appearing in the July/August 2002 issue of *Psychosomatic Medicine* found that coffee drinking is harder on the body than we may have thought. James D. Lane, Ph.D., associate research professor in the Department of Psychiatry and Behavioral Sciences at Duke asserted, "The effects of coffee drinking are long-lasting and exaggerate the stress response both in terms of the body's physiological response in blood pressure elevations and stress hormone levels, but it also magnifies a person's perception of stress. Dr. Lane goes on to explain, "Our evidence, and that of other studies, shows that this downside exists and people should be aware of it in order to make the best possible health choices."

During the study conducted at Duke, coffee drinkers wore a portable monitor that measured blood pressure and heart rate and tracked statistics four times an hour from early morning until bedtime, while they went about their normal daily activities. Participants collected urine samples so that the researchers could measure the amount of stress hormones they had produced that day. They were also asked to keep a diary to record their perceived stress levels as well as their physical position—standing, sitting or lying down—each time the monitor was activated.

When the researchers compared the caffeine days to the placebo days they discovered that caffeine consumption significantly raised blood pressure throughout the day and night, and adrenaline levels rose by 32 percent. The researchers found that the elevated levels stayed elevated through to bedtime.

The study also demonstrated that caffeine appears to compound the effects of stress both psychologically in terms of perceived stress levels and in terms of elevated blood pressures and stress hormone levels, as if the stressor is actually of greater magnitude. The combination of stress and caffeine has a multiplying, or synergistically negative effect. Not good.

The researchers noted that while habitual coffee drinkers might be expected to demonstrate tolerance to the effects of caffeine, they still showed significant responses to the drug. The researchers said that despite the assumed safety of overwhelmingly popular caffeinated beverages such as coffee, the caffeine drug does show short-term negative health effects that, if continued over a period of years, could increase the risk of heart attack and stroke.

If that is not enough, Duke University also conducted a study that has been replicated numerous times that indicated a strong correlation between caffeine intake and breast pain and the incidence of fibrocystic breasts. This study supports the findings of others in that caffeine restriction is an effective means of management of breast pain associated with fibrocystic disease.

So caffeine is bad? What about decaffeinated coffee? Many health conditions that are aggravated by coffee are still affected by decaffeinated coffee, despite the lowered level of caffeine, due to these other phytochemicals that remain in decaf coffee after the decaffeination process. Current studies suggest that for people who are sensitive to coffee's effects, decaffeinated brews may still exacerbate their health problems. Therefore, the healthiest option may be to eliminate both regular and decaffeinated coffee from the diet.

The decaffeination process itself is not always innocuous. There are two common decaffeination methods: 1) The use of solvents, either methylene chloride or ethyl acetate, is used in 80 percent of decaffeinated coffees. The health effects of these solvents as found in decaffeinated coffee are not well known, but studies suggest that methylene chloride (dichloromethane) is shown to be carcinogenic. In the decaffeination process, the solvents are removed from the coffee beans, but residues have still been found in decaffeinated coffee and tea. 2) Water extraction, also known as the Swiss water process or European water process, and supercritical carbon dioxide are the two other processes. When water and carbon dioxide are used to decaffeinate coffee, a measurable residue is not left behind in the remaining beans, but high acidity and other phytochemicals found in coffee do remain.

According to FDA guidelines, decaffeinated coffee must have 97 percent of the caffeine removed. In actuality, the caffeine content of coffee beans varies widely; therefore the caffeine content of decaffeinated coffee also fluctuates, and can be 10mg or more per 12-ounce cup.

Most decaffeinated coffee is made from Robusta beans. Robusta beans are used because they retain more of the coffee flavor after the decaffeination process. Ironically, Robusta beans have a higher concentration of caffeine and are more acidic than other beans. This is problematic for people with health problems such as acid reflux, GERD and ulcers. In essence, the seemingly healthier choice of a decaffeinated coffee makes these people even more susceptible to the detrimental effects of high levels of acidity.

Additionally, levels of LDL cholesterol, a strong predictor for heart disease, have been shown to increase after coffee drinkers switch from regular coffee to decaf coffee. The results of these studies suggest that other components in coffee, not removed in the decaffeination process, are responsible for increasing the risk factors for heart disease. Decaf coffee has also been shown to raise plasma levels of homocysteine, which is associated with increased susceptibility of developing cardiovascular disease due to the levels of chlorogenic acid.

Just like regular coffee, decaf coffee stimulates the sympathetic or autonomic nervous system, which raises heart rate, blood pressure and causes the shaking and tremors that are commonly thought of as "coffee jitters." Decaf coffee can cause laxative effects similar to regular coffee in spite of the reduced amount of caffeine. Decaf coffee interferes with the absorption of minerals such as iron, calcium and magnesium.

Coffee, even decaffeinated, stimulates the sympathetic (fight or flight) nervous system regardless of the amount of caffeine present. Increased heart rate, arterial blood pressure and muscle sympathetic nervous activity, including hand shaking, tremors or jitters are all stimulated by decaffeinated as well as regular coffee, indicating that it is a substance other than caffeine present in coffee creating these effects.

Both decaffeinated and regular coffee cause similar increases in gastroesopheal sphincter pressure making GERD symptoms worse, while pressure changed minimally in response to pure caffeine, tap water or black (caffeinated) tea. This indicates that compounds in coffee other than caffeine are responsible for increased incidence of acid reflux after coffee consumption.

Now, in the effort of fairness, coffee has also been shown to have positive affect on athletic performance given at the right quantity before exercise in athletes including strenuous activities such as sprinting and competitive sports.

Probably the best kept secret about coffee is that it delivers more antioxidants than even green tea. Green coffee beans contain about 1,000 antioxidants, and the brewing process adds 300 more. The roasting process, by the way, creates its own set of healthful compounds which, like some antioxidants, are unique to coffee alone.

Three major, long-term studies, as well as numerous smaller studies, have confirmed coffee's properties for preventing type 2, or "adult-onset," diabetes.

A powerful antioxidant found almost exclusively in coffee, methylpyridinium, boosts blood enzymes widely believed to protect against colon cancer. Coffee enemas have been a standard method of detox for the liver and colon for hundreds of years.

Results also suggested that unique coffee compounds contribute to the beneficial effect. Other caffeinated beverages did not offer the same level of protection, and decaffeinated coffee provided lesser protection, while decaffeinated tea offered none.

So now what do you do? Coffee is both bad for you and good for you! Well, this is a prime example of the uniqueness of the science of nutrition. What is one person's food is another's poison. In no other science do you find two equally good studies showing exactly opposite results. Why? Each person is biochemically unique. For some people, coffee is an elixir; for others it is not.

What I have found is that many of The Cleanse Program participants were addicted to caffeine, which means that they were consuming too much. So, to bring you back into balance, we will be cutting out coffee during The Cleanse Program.

Don't worry hard core coffee addicts. On the cleanse, you will be slowly reducing coffee intake by switching to green and black tea which contain antioxidants and much lower levels of caffeine. By the end of the cleanse, you will find that getting completely off coffee will actually increase your energy and may even reduce some symptoms you have been living with such as elevated blood pressure, stress and elevated cholesterol.

ALCOHOL APPREHENSIONS

Alcohol, or ethyl alcohol (ethanol), is the intoxicating ingredient found in wine, beer and hard liquor. Alcohol is created when the carbohydrates in grains, fruits, and vegetables are combined with micro-organisms. The combination of yeast or bacteria and carbohydrates causes fermentation that produces the by-product "alcohol." Alcohol is not on The Cleanse Program.

Every alcoholic beverage has different amounts of alcohol. The amount of alcohol in distilled liquor is known as "proof." Proof refers to the amount of alcohol in the liquor. For example, 100-proof liquor contains 50 percent alcohol and 40-proof liquor contains 20 percent alcohol, and so on.

How the Body Metabolizes Alcohol

Because alcohol requires no digestion, the body is able to metabolize it extremely quickly taking it straight to the blood stream from the small intestines and liver for detoxification. About 20 percent is absorbed directly through the walls of an empty stomach and can reach the brain within only one minute. In addition, about 10 percent of the alcohol is expelled through the breath and urine.

Once alcohol reaches the stomach, it begins to break down with the alcohol dehydrogenase enzyme. This process reduces the amount of alcohol entering the blood by approximately 20 percent. Some people are actually genetically incapable of producing this enzyme. Generally speaking, women produce less of this enzyme, which may help to explain why women become more intoxicated with less alcohol than men.

Alcohol is rapidly absorbed in the upper portion of the small intestine. The alcohol-laden blood then travels to the liver via the veins and capillaries of the digestive tract, which affects nearly every liver cell. The liver cells are the only cells in our body that can produce enough of the enzyme alcohol dehydrogenase to oxidize alcohol at an appreciable rate.

Though alcohol affects every organ of the body, its most dramatic impact is upon the liver. Liver cells normally prefer fatty acids as fuel. Excess acids are packaged as triglycerides, which then route to other tissues of the body. However, when alcohol is present, the liver cells are forced to first metabolize the alcohol. The fatty acids accumulate, sometimes in large amounts in the liver. Alcohol metabolism permanently transforms liver cell structure and impairs the liver's ability to metabolize fats. This explains why heavy drinkers tend to develop fatty livers.

The liver is able to metabolize about one-half an ounce of ethanol per hour (approximately one drink, depending on a person's body size, food intake, etc.). If more alcohol is consumed, the liver enzymes become overrun and the excess alcohol travels to all parts of the body, circulating until the liver enzymes are finally able to process it. This is the reason for the intoxicating affect of alcohol.

How the Liver Processes Alcohol

The alcohol dehydrogenase enzyme deconstructs alcohol by removing hydrogen. First, the alcohol dehydrogenase oxidizes alcohol to acetaldehyde, which is then acted on by the acetaldehyde dehydrogenase enzyme creating acetaldehyde to acetyl CoA. These reactions produce hydrogen ions (acid). The B vitamin niacin (in its role as the coenzyme NAD) picks up these hydrogen ions and becomes NADH.

When alcohol is metabolized, NAD (Nicotinamide adenine dinucleotide) diminishes and NADH (Nicotinamide adenine dinucleotide dehydrogenase) increases. During alcohol metabolism, NAD becomes unavailable for the many other vital body processes for which it is needed, including: Glycolysis: breakdown of glucose, The TCA (Citric Acid Cycle) and the electron transport chain, which is part of the metabolic pathway that converts fats, carbohydrates and proteins to energy.

Without NAD, the energy pathway is blocked, and alternative measures are taken by the body that cause an accumulation of hydrogen atoms which shifts the body's balance toward acidic.

The accumulation of NADH slows the TCA, resulting in a buildup of pyruvate (a by-product of glucose metabolism) and acetyl CoA (molecule created when carbon atoms are oxidized for energy production). Excess acetyl CoA results in fatty acid synthesis and fat begins to clog the liver. Incidentally, an accumulation of fat in the liver can be observed after only a single night of heavy drinking. By the way, fructose and especially high fructose corn syrup metabolizes the same way except you do not get the buzz as you would from alcohol.

Fatty Liver and Liver Disease

With moderate drinking (see below for definition), the liver can process alcohol fairly safely. However, heavy drinking overburdens the liver resulting in fat accumulation in the liver. A clogged, fatty liver causes liver cells to become less efficient at performing their necessary tasks, resulting in impairment of a person's nutritional health. Fatty liver is the first stage of liver damage in heavy drinkers, and interferes with the supply of oxygen and nutrients to the liver's cells. If liver damage continues, the liver cells will die, forming fibrous scar tissue called fibrosis. The last stage of deterioration is called cirrhosis and is the least reversible. Some liver cells can regenerate with good nutrition and abstinence; however, the more damage done to the liver, the less possibility for recovery.

Alcohol and Malnutrition

For moderate drinkers, alcohol may actually increase appetite and reduce inhibition leading to poor food choices. However, chronic alcohol consumption appears to have the opposite effect.

Alcohol is calorie dense, packing seven calories per gram. But like pure sugar, the calories are void of nutrients. To make matters worse, chronic alcohol abuse not only disrupts appetite, but also interferes with the body's ability to metabolize nutrients. This interference causes damage to the liver, digestive system and nearly every organ.

Heavy alcohol consumption with a decrease in appetite increases the risk of protein malnutrition and low intakes of the following: protein, calcium, iron, vitamin A, vitamin C, thiamine, vitamin B6 and riboflavin. Absorption of calcium, phosphorus, vitamin D and zinc are also impaired.

To Drink or Not to Drink?

Recent studies indicate that moderate use of alcohol may have a beneficial effect on the coronary system. In general, for healthy people, one drink per day for women and no more than two drinks per day for men should be considered the maximum amount of alcohol consumption to be considered moderate use. However, the amount of alcohol that a person can drink safely is highly individual, depending on genetics, age, sex, weight and family history.

A "drink" is considered to be:

- 4–5-ounces of wine
- 10-ounces of wine cooler
- 12-ounces of beer

    1–1 ¼-ounces of distilled liquor (80-proof whiskey, vodka, scotch or rum)

5
A Peek in the Pantry

> *The correlation between poverty and obesity can be traced to agricultural policies and subsidies.*
> *– Michael Pollan, author of* The Omnivore's Dilemma

In the early 1900s, farmers represented 40 percent of the American population. Our nation consisted of farms that ranged in size from small family farms to commercial production farms. Today, less than 10 percent of Americans are farmers, and the American farm has grown in size by over 40 percent on average. Our national source of nutritional and energetic intake has become big business. Small farms cater to consumer needs; big, commercial farms cater to, and answer to, Wall Street.

As we mindlessly gaze into our refrigerators and pantries, mindfully prepare a family meal, or walk the aisles of the supermarket selecting items to place in our shopping cart, we are actively participating in the intricately detailed and overwhelmingly confusing industry known as agribusiness. A peek in the pantry is a peek into a trillion dollar business that involves many industries—farmers, chemical engineers, transportation, retail, advertising, marketing, public relations, finance, product package manufacturing, political lobbying and many more—all with the goal of getting the consumer (i.e., you) to buy more product. The food industry's goal is to sell product not to promote wellness or preserve health.

BS IN MARKETING

The United States is a nation of agricultural abundance. American farms produce enough food to feed every American twice over. In an industry as saturated with available nutritional resources as the American food industry is, corporations must encourage consumers to buy, and eat, more and more product in order to stay profitable and keep shareholders happy. In her book, *The Politics Of Food*, Marion Nestle explains how the food industry tackles this ever-increasing "problem" of selling more food in the land of agricultural plenty. Corporations must determine what the consumer wants, which includes developing campaigns to persuade the consumer to "want" what the food industry has a plethora of (i.e., corn, soy and wheat), in order to make a profit. Nutritional content is taken into consideration only when it is necessary to entice buyers. For example, products marketed as "low carb" flew off the shelves at the height of the Atkin's diet mania, regardless of whether or not a high protein/low-carbohydrate diet was indeed healthful.

While we all would like to think that we are unaffected by marketing ploys or advertising campaigns, we are not. We are all influenced by our surroundings and the onslaught of information overload presented in our daily lives from digital media, to print media, to subliminal messaging in the form of sounds, temperature, lighting and product display at the supermarket. And while some product messaging is blatant, most is not.

Nestle identifies four factors that drive all marketing initiatives in the food industry: taste, cost, convenience and public confusion. Most western cultures have developed a taste for foods that are sweet, salty and fatty in flavor. We tend to select foods that fit in with our cultural understanding of familiarity in terms of flavor, texture, smell and aesthetics—how the food looks. Much research is conducted to isolate preferential tastes of groups of people in terms of age, education, gender, geographical locations, income levels and ethnic background. Every product on the supermarket shelf has passed rigorous market tests, undergone extensive market research and has highly specified shelf placement. In the food industry, nothing is left to chance.

Americans are a highly cost-conscious society, especially when it comes to our food. Most Americans will sacrifice nutrition in order to save money, and the food industry is acutely aware of this characteristic in the collective personality of the American consumer. The more processed the food, the less nutritive the product. The longer the shelf life, the lower cost per unit the food manufacturer can offer the product and still receive the highest profit margin per unit—a seemingly win-win for both the consumer and the corporation. Except, of course, the consumer loses big in terms of nutrition and healthful benefits of the food. While cost plays an imperative role in marketing for the food manufacturer, it is the consumer's responsibility to make healthy and smart buying decisions.

Convenience has become an American value. We are a fast-paced society, and big agribusiness knows that. Campbell's Soup® makes a soup packaged in a cup—just pop it in the microwave and go. McDonald's provides salad in a cup to appeal to the mom or dad who wants to eat a "healthy" meal in the car while feeding the children Happy Meals®. Slim Fast® makes drinking your dinner quick and easy. Many food manufacturers have a 100-calorie snack pack—a genius marketing ploy. Convenience has become next to godliness. Once again, profit margins are tied closely to the convenience that is "sold" as a lifestyle solution. Highly processed food void of nutrients is the price many Americans are willing to pay for this convenience.

Public confusion is another highly effective marketing strategy of big agribusiness. Eat carbs—don't eat carbs; eat high a protein diet—too much protein is toxic; eat a non-fat diet—our bodies require fat in order to lose weight; eat six to eight small meals throughout the day—don't eat after six in the evening. Understanding what to eat, when to eat it and in what form to eat it has become something in which entire academic and professional industries have sprouted. And, with all the professionals and academics providing well-researched and seemingly unbiased information, the general public remains more confused than ever. As consumers, we receive most of our nutritional education through the advertising and marketing campaigns of large, food corporations. We are not receiving objective information. For example, most people do not understand the terms organic, natural, all-natural and 100 percent natural or the difference between free-range and grass-fed, and that is no accident. Much of the information we receive regarding nutrition, we read about in various forms of media, the Internet or learn about through television advertising campaigns, the news and "special" reports. But much of this information is generated from research, studies, experts and public relations representatives paid for by food corporations seeking a nutritional slant to a new product or a product they are seeking to revive.

There is nothing more dangerous to the food industry than a well-educated consumer. Just about every food and beverage manufacturer has a top public relations firm and a trade association tasked at promoting the benefits of the product in a way that speaks to its intended audience and gets the media's, professionals' and consumers' "buy-in" on the value of buying and consuming the product. These public relation firms and trade associations are not just lobbying the consumers, they are lobbying congress as well for how the message can and cannot be presented to the consumer.

When we take a peek in the pantry, we take a peek at the powerful world of marketing. We also take a peek at the power of politics.

POLITICS IN THE PANTRY

American consumers have a tendency to trust that the government is serving as an honest, objective and unbiased consumer watchdog. We believe that if the Federal Food and Drug Agency has given its stamp of approval, these foods are either good for us or at the very least not harmful. Unfortunately, this is not the case.

Walk through any grocery store, and you will be bombarded with health and ingredient claims written in bold on the front of their packaging: Reduces Cholesterol, Boosts Immunity, No Trans Fats! Wow, all I need is some cereal and my cholesterol will go down to normal; I will never get sick, and I do not have to worry about inflammation from bad fats! I guess all of the whole foods that make up the perimeter of the store are just unnecessary. Your mom probably told you not to believe everything you read. In this case, she was absolutely correct.

Where did all of these healthcare claims come from?

In 1997 the Quaker Oats Company asked the FDA to approve a health message for their cereal label, letting consumers know that a diet rich in soluble fiber found in oatmeal and low in fat may reduce the risk of heart disease. After reviewing the single scientific study on oatmeal showing a minor reduction in cholesterol, the agency green-lighted the health claim. The new health claim pasted on those old-fashioned, rounded oatmeal canisters reversed a major slump in sales. Amazing!

How does a health claim get assigned to a product?

According to the FDA Web site, "Claims that can be used on food and dietary supplement labels fall into three categories: health claims, nutrient content claims, and structure/function claims. The responsibility for ensuring the validity of these claims rests with the manufacturer, FDA, or, in the case of advertising, with the Federal Trade Commission."

So how are these claims defined?

Health claims are used to describe a relationship between a food, a food component or a supplement ingredient and the action of reducing the risk of a disease or health-related condition. The following are the three ways in which the FDA oversees health claims on a label or in labeling for a food or dietary supplement.

In the 1990 Nutrition Labeling and Education Act (NLEA), the FDA issued regulations authorizing health claims for foods and dietary supplements after an FDA review of the scientific evidence submitted in a health claim petition created by the manufacturer.

The 1997 Food and Drug Administration Modernization Act (FDAMA) allowed for health claims based on an authoritative statement from a scientific organization of the U.S. government or the National Academy of Sciences. These claims may be used after submitting a health claim notification to the FDA.

A "health claim" has two essential components: 1) a substance (whether a food, a food component or ingredient) and 2) a disease or health-related condition. A statement missing either one of these pieces does not meet the regulatory definition of a health claim. According to the FDA, dietary guidance statements used on food labels must be truthful and non-misleading.

FDA authorizes these types of health claims based on a review of the scientific literature, generally as a result of the submission of a health claim petition by a manufacturer. If the evidence for a particular claim is not well established, qualifying language is included as part of the claim to indicate that the evidence supporting the claim is limited. So the claim can still be made with a notation that the claim has not been supported by the FDA. If you would like a good example of this, the nutritional supplement industry is able to make claims but must note that the claims have not been subject to FDA approval.

Sounds like a manufacturer can make a claim even if the FDA does not support it, right? Or is that what it means? Is this confusing to you? It is confusing to the entire U.S. population! The FDA has even conducted a study regarding the food packages in grocery stores. The study examines claims about health, and the FDA found that consumers are confused by what they are reading. The confusion began escalating in 2002, which is when the FDA added a whole new category of approved claims. These are called qualified claims, statements that are backed by some evidence but lack scientific consensus.

The 2003 FDA Consumer Health Information for Better Nutrition Initiative had provisions for qualified health claims where the quality and strength of the scientific evidence falls below that required for FDA to issue what they call an authorizing regulation. These health claims are supposed to be qualified to assure accuracy and make sure it is not misleading to consumers.

A "structure and function" claim may not imply that a disease or health-related condition is related to a food, a food component or ingredient. These claims have historically appeared on the labels used by processed foods and dietary supplements as well as drugs. Structure and function claims describe the role of a nutrient or dietary ingredient intended to affect normal structure or function in humans such as "fiber increases bowel regularity."

Structure/function claims may also describe a benefit related to a nutrient deficiency disease such as scurvy and vitamin C as long as the statement also informs the consumer about how widespread such a disease is in the United States. The manufacturer is responsible for ensuring the accuracy and truthfulness of these claims; they are not pre-approved by the FDA, but the claims must be truthful and not misleading. If a dietary supplement label includes such a claim, it must state in a "disclaimer" that the FDA has not evaluated the claim. The disclaimer must also state that the dietary supplement product is not intended to "diagnose, treat, cure or prevent any disease," because only a drug can legally make such a claim even though many drugs mechanism of action mimics the action of natural herbs and nutrients found in nature. For instance, Red Yeast Rice has been used for thousands of years in Chinese medicine. The major active constituent, monacolin K in red yeast rice, is the same as lovastatin, an active ingredient in the cholesterol-lowering drug, MEVACOR®. A number of clinical trials have demonstrated effectiveness in using red yeast rice preparations for reducing cholesterol levels in high cholesterol patients.

The Nutrition Labeling and Education Act of 1990 (NLEA) permits the use of claims that characterize the level of a particular nutrient in a food such as sodium. Nutrient content claims describe the level of a nutrient or dietary substance in the product, using terms such as "free, high and low," or they compare the level of a nutrient in a food to that of another food, using terms such as "more, reduced and light." Most nutrient content claim regulations apply only to those nutrients or dietary substances that have an established daily minimum value.

So what are the common labels gracing the processed foods in our grocery stores?

- Sugar Free: This often screams, "artificial sweeteners added." So make sure you know which ones they are. Artificial sweeteners are worse than real sugar. It also could mean that fruits or fruit juice was added.

- Low Fat: The food has less than three grams of fat per serving. Most of the time, when fat is removed from a food, sugar or refined starches have been used to replace the fat to keep it palatable. This is also true of other low fat claims such as "light" (50 percent less fat), "fat free" (less than one gram of fat) and reduced fat (25 percent less fat). Often, these abominations can be worse than their higher fat counterparts and may also be similar or higher in calories (sugar calories).

- Zero-Grams (0) Trans-Fats: When you see this, bet money there are trans fats in the product. It means that there is less than a gram per serving or up to 500mg per serving. Look for the words "No Trans Fats."
- Low Carb: Foods that are not normally low in carbohydrates, such as bread or candy, are made to be low carb by replacing the carbohydrate component with fiber, artificial sweeteners and sugar alcohols.
- All Natural: This claim means nothing. Manufacturers are allowed to put this on practically any food without any proof of anything.
- Corn-Fed/Vegetarian-Fed/Grain-Fed/Grain-Finished Beef: This label is supposed to make you feel as though you are getting high-quality beef and implies that the cow was eating what it would naturally eat. Do not be fooled. Cattle were never meant to eat corn. Cattle get very sick when they eat corn and are fed antibiotics to counteract the infections created by the faulty grain diet. Look for 100 percent grass-fed beef.
- USDA Organic: Now we are talking! This is the only health claim with teeth. The food industry is attempting to lessen restrictions on what "organic" means and allow non-organic processes under the organic label. It means no pesticides, no herbicides, no antibiotics and no chemicals. Period. What constitutes organic meats, fowl and fish is very strict. The animals' feed must be free of chemicals: no hormones or antibiotics can be given to the animals. The organic claim does not, however, guarantee the animals are treated better than their factory-farmed counterparts. And, "organic" in no way implies "grass-fed." Unless it implicitly states, "grass-fed," assume the cow or chicken was fed organic corn.
- Access to Pasture and Free-Range: Ah, animals frolicking in the countryside enjoying life. Not exactly. This misleading label has no requirements and does not have any regulations. It really has relatively little meaning, and it can consist of a little more than an hour in a pen outside or so called "access" to the outside such as a window in the barn. The only way to know for sure if the animal is free range is to visit the farm—the actual farm, not their Web site.

If we synthetically fortify foods with basic building block vitamins, then we will have healthy diets, right? This is a dangerous way to think; every year there are new things we never knew we could not live without: lycopene, antioxidants, resveratrol and the list goes on. Just look at the grocery store shelves. The antithesis to reductionist nutrition is eating a variety of fresh foods, mostly plants.

So what does this all mean to you? It is real simple. The foods that have the most nutrients, antioxidants, vitamins and minerals are the ones without labels: vegetables, fruits, legumes, whole grains, dairy, eggs, meats, fish and fowl. These foods do not need labels with fancy, albeit dubious, claims about nutrient content.

The real fact is that all foods that are processed—changed from how they grow on the planet into something else (e.g., brown rice to Rice Krispies)—and lose their nutrients in the refining and manufacturing process. These foods are then enriched (adding back the nutrients removed during processing) to have some nutrient value. Most of the grocery store is filled with nutrient-poor, calorie dense foods in which the food manufacturers are grabbing at straws to try and get you to buy.

The lesson? Do not judge a food by its wrapper! Here is a great rule to live by: The more marketing, advertising and endorsements a food product has is inversely proportional to the nutritive value of the food. If a celebrity promotes it in a commercial, and it is always on the header at a grocery store, the food has little food value. When possible avoid the wrapper all together.

The food industry has influenced what Americans eat through lobbying, advertising and aggressive maneuvering around legislation. According to Marion Nestle, the U.S. government has gone from urging Americans to eat more, to curbing their consumption in a matter of decades. This has led food producers and manufacturers to market their products through lobbying of the FDA and aiming at specific consumer groups, most notably children.

The food industry has a very basic goal: to sell as much food as possible. This goal can only lead to consumers eating more. So on one hand the U.S. government is charged with influencing the economy and bolstering the American bottom line, and on the other hand, we expect the government to provide guidelines for eating well. In a very fundamental way, these two expectations are decidedly at odds.

As consumers, we need to understand why and how our government is so adept at confusing us about diet and health issues. Promoting confusion is especially costly the sick-care costs (healthcare costs) are escalating out of sight (The U.S. has highest per capita costs in the world.), health care quality is declining (The U.S. is ranked 37th in the world.) and shorter life spans are now being projected.

Few, if any, explanations of this on-going tragedy are more important than our misunderstanding of the ability of nutrition to help maintain health. But being confused about nutrition is not surprising. We just can't help it. Government funding for nutrition research and education is almost non-existent. According to Nestle's, *Food Politics*, the food industry has incredible political clout using lobbying procedures to gain government support, increasing the ability to market junk foods as health foods and the use of false or misleading food claims. Through the inappropriate use of power, we can begin to understand how the American population is confused, and where the breach between what consumers are supposed to eat and what they actually do eat has occurred.

During Ronald Reagan's tenure as president, the USDA moved ketchup from what it truly is—a sugar-laden condiment—to being considered a vegetable. Today, potatoes (a concentrated starch), corn (another starch) and ketchup (sugar) are the three top consumed "vegetables" by children in the United States. First, do you think that determining whether ketchup is worthy as a vegetable is good use of the government's time and resources? Second, what? Ketchup, really? Give me a break. Children are the unfortunate targets of countless numbers of snack campaigns, which only serve to further the obesity epidemic. For the record, ketchup is concentrated high-fructose corn syrup with tomatoes waved over it.

The United Stated Department of Agriculture (USDA) has repeatedly shown that it is more interested in the economy of the U.S. agriculture industry than in the health of the taxpaying American citizens. The majority of the members involved in creating the most recent USDA approved food pyramid had unrevealed conflicts of interest with the dairy industry that only became known through a court order. From the perspective of the USDA, politics, economics, and money matter more than the health of the American people.

HOW BIG FARM IS KILLING US!

It is important for American consumers to know the "life cycle" of our food. Author, journalist and advocate for real foods, Michael Pollan, has written numerous books detailing the history of food in the United States as well as the life cycle of food in the Standard American Diet. In his book, *The Omnivore's Dilemma,* Pollan details all aspects of food: production, consumption, evolution, emotion, health, community, environment and philosophy. Pollan discusses how corn has become the central player in our modern industrial food production. Corn, or some corn by-product, has worked its way into almost every processed food item that we eat, including most of the beef sold in the United States. If you add wheat, wheat by-products and soy, you have the primary ingredients in almost every processed food.

Much of the meat products we consume from restaurants, supermarkets and fast foods today come from feedlots where calves spend their last days getting fattened up on corn and antibiotics. Residence on the feedlot is relatively short-lived for most cattle. They consume copious amounts of corn and antibiotics in order for them to be delivered to the slaughterhouse nice and fat. Corn-fed beef is a relatively new invention that requires a veterinary staff armed with concoction of drugs to implement.

So what are factory farms, CAFOs (Confined Animal Feeding Operation) and feedlots? They are giant livestock "farms" that house thousands of cows, chickens or pigs in confined pens where these animals stand around in their own excrement eating corn out of troughs. Chickens are often kept in cages with so many in one cage they are pressed tightly against and on top of one another. Pens confining pigs and cows are often so overcrowded that the animals cannot move freely. Theses "animal farms" produce staggering amounts of animal wastes.

On most factory farms, the excrement is funneled into massive waste lagoons or pools. These toxic pools often leak or overflow, sending dangerous microbes, nitrate pollution and drug-resistant bacteria into our nation's water supplies. The food borne contamination of spinach in 2006 was tied to run-off from factory farms contaminating farm water with E.coli.

Factory farms and toxic lagoons also emit toxic gases such as ammonia, hydrogen sulfide and methane. Additionally, the farms spray the manure onto land, ostensibly as fertilizer bringing still more of these harmful substances into the air and water. Emissions of these gases have been tied to asthma, breathing difficulties and illnesses in children and adults living in close proximity to the CAFO.

Oddly enough, in spite of the huge amounts of animal waste that factory farms produce, they have largely escaped pollution regulations; loopholes and weak enforcement share the blame. Now, the U.S. Environmental Protection Agency (EPA) is under court order to set tighter controls on the release of pathogens such E.Coli found in cattle excrement into the environment by factory farms, exercise greater oversight on factory farms and ensure that these plans are made available to the public.

These types of operations are a threat to human health. People who live near or work at CAFOs breathe in toxic gasses, which are formed as manure decomposes. The stink can be unbearable; but even worse, the harmful gasses released by the lagoons, such as hydrogen sulfide, which is dangerous even at low levels, permeate the air. The toxic waste pools also contaminate drinking water supplies. Several disease and food contamination outbreaks related to drinking water have been traced to bacteria and viruses from waste.

In addition, the truckloads of antibiotics also pose dangers. CAFOs routinely give animals antibiotics to compensate for illness resulting from the crowded conditions and unnatural diet. These antibiotics are entering the environment and the food chain, contributing to the rise of antibiotic-resistant bacteria and making it harder to treat infectious diseases.

The United States water quality is threatened by phosphorus and nitrogen, two nutrients present in animal waste. In excessive amounts, phosphorous and nitrogen can cause an explosion of algae that robs oxygen from the water, killing aquatic life. So when we have run-off, we destroy our rivers, oceans, lakes and oceans.

As consumers, we have the power to change the way our food is produced. Our power is easy to exercise and requires only small lifestyle changes. We do not need to start a political lobbying or action group. All we have to do is place our vote utilizing our debit, credit cards and checkbooks. If we refuse to support the feedlots financially, they will be forced to change. The good news is that it only takes about a 10 percent shift in spending patterns to change an industry.

One example of the almighty dollar's ability to create change occurred in the dairy industry. In the not too distant past, recumbant bovine somatotropin (rBST) was used in large amounts in the U.S. to improve dairy production yield (increase milk production) in cows. Consumers decided they did not want to ingest large amounts of bovine hormones in their dairy products. With the rapid, albeit relatively small, change in public opinion, almost overnight the use of rBST dropped to next to none in the United States. Consumers began buying rBST-free dairy and the industry changed in order to retain their customers.

As consumers, we hold power over the food industry; all it takes is conscious spending. In the grocery store, this means checking labels for "organic," "free range" (remember to do your homework to verify the free-range claim), "antibiotic-free" or similar wording that indicates meat that was raised in a more sustainable manner. Another option is to support sustainable livestock farms that sell directly to consumers or through local farmers' markets. We have the power to change the world, one dollar at a time.

GENETICALLY MODIFIED FOODS

Why should we care about genetically modified foods? Genetic engineering of crops is a complex and controversial issue. GM crops are untested and have already been implicated in several far-reaching environmental and health-related tragedies such as the relationship between GM Bt corn pollen and the declining population of Monarch butterflies and other animal species. Genetically modified food has far-reaching implications for the environment and for people, for the way crops are produced and the way the world's people are fed.

The introduction of GM crops increases the pressure on already damaged and vulnerable environments and has failed to decrease the use of insecticides and herbicides, one of the many assumed benefits from the process. A sustainable approach to agriculture that is environmentally, economically, culturally and socially responsible helps to protect the environment and improve food quality. Growing genetically modified crops does the opposite.

People have been selectively breeding or crossbreeding plants for centuries. For example, plants have been crossbred to adapt them to a particular climate or to improve their yield. What makes genetic engineering radically different from traditional breeding methods is that genes are transferred between completely unrelated species. For instance, animal genes are transferred to plants and bacteria genes are moved across to food crops. So, your next corn chip may, and probably does, contain genes from bacteria.

Types of genetically modified crops:

- Insecticide crops: These have had genes transferred from a natural bacterium so that they can act like insecticide plants and kill the pests that eat them.

- Roundup® Ready crops (the brainchild of Monsanto): These crops are tolerant to specific herbicides. When these herbicides are applied, only weeds and non-Roundup® plants are killed. The Roundup® Ready plants are preserved.

- Other GM crops include those that have been made resistant to fungal infections and those that have had their nutritional properties enhanced such as "golden rice," which contains vitamin A.

Advocates of genetically modified crops argue that GM crops are good for the environment since they reduce the amount of pesticides and herbicides used in crop production. However, this has proven to be a failed assumption. Now, after over 10 years of producing genetically modified crops, insecticides and herbicide usage on GM crops has increased significantly. They require fewer chemicals than conventional crops in the short term, but over time they require significantly more.

Genetically modified organisms (GMOs) threaten plant biodiversity. Planting GM crops is not a question of choice: Once they are planted, neighboring crops become contaminated via cross-pollination. This is especially disastrous for organic farmers. For example, although it is illegal to grow genetically modified corn in Mexico, in 2001 researchers found that traditional corn varieties grown by farmers in two remote Mexican states were contaminated with GMOs from GM corn. There are thousands of varieties of corn in Mexico. If all of these varieties become contaminated by GMOs, these precious indigenous varieties could become extinct.

Some farmers whose conventional crops have been contaminated by genetically modified material have found themselves heavily fined by biotech corporations (that own the patented GM material) for the natural process of cross-pollination. Biotech companies are also quite litigious and have been actively suing small farmers in court, tying up years of court time and costing the farmer extraordinary amounts of money to defend themselves. Farmers are being sued for having GMOs on their property that they did not buy, do not want, will not use and cannot sell, all because a GMO corn kernel fell on their land and sprouted.

Genetically modified crops are produced for corporate profit, not to feed the hungry or to improve the environment. Genetically modified seeds are patented (naturally obtained seeds cannot be patented) and strictly controlled by the biotech companies. The seeds and the chemicals (herbicides and pesticides) that are required to grow these genetically modified seeds must be purchased from the multinational biotech corporations. Farmers are prohibited from saving and sharing seeds—a time honored, farming tradition. Every year farmers must buy more seeds and the associated chemicals from the corporations.

GMOs have been under fire in Europe and in several developing countries such as Angola, India, Sudan, Zambia and Malawi. All of these countries have said no to genetically modified crops. They have also resisted GM foods as food aid. The United States Agency for International Development (USAID) has exerted enormous pressure through the United Nations World Food Program, effectively telling countries that they have no choice: accept GM food, or get no food aid at all. The GM bumper crops being grown in the U.S. have to go somewhere.

What is the alternative to genetically modified agriculture? Sustainable agriculture is environmentally, economically, culturally and socially sustainable. Sustainable agriculture emphasizes crop diversity and rotation, conserves natural resources such as soil quality and mineral content, and favors small and medium-sized farming rather than large agribusinesses and large corporations. Moreover, sustainable agriculture focuses on food variety prioritizing the production of staple crops rather than cash crops for export.

There are a number of dangers associated with consuming genetically modified foods that broadly fall into the categories of potential toxins, allergens, carcinogens, new diseases, antibiotic resistant diseases and nutritional problems. Much of the details of these potential dangers have been meticulously documented in the books, *Seeds of Deception* and *Genetic Roulette: The Documented Health Risks of Genetically Engineered Foods* by Jeffery Smith. I highly recommend reading both.

Research does not point to the safety of consuming genetically modified foods. Only one feeding study has been conducted with humans, and it showed that GMOs survive inside the stomach of the people eating GMO food. No follow-up studies have been conducted. Several animal feeding studies have shown GMOs to potentially be correlated with pre-cancerous cell growth, damaged immune systems, decreased brain size, testicular changes, liver damage, partial destruction or increased density of the liver, false pregnancies and higher death rates.

An additional concern regarding genetically modified foods is that the technology to test whether there are in fact chemical differences between GM foods and non-GM foods at the DNA level has yet to be developed. The biotech industry supports the idea that we have been consuming genetically modified foods without ill effect. However, there is no governing body investigating the effects of GM foods on humans. Moreover, it might take years or decades before we see the full effect of GM foods on the population. There are some organizations that believe GM foods may be playing a role in the increase of food allergies in the human population. According to Jeffery Smith, after GM soy was introduced to the United Kingdom, soy allergies increased by a full 50 percent.

Still not convinced? In March 2001, the Center for Disease Control (CDC) reported that food is responsible for two times the number of illnesses in the U.S. compared to estimates from just seven years ago. Coincidence? I think not. This increase corresponds to the period in which Americans began unknowingly eating GM food.

Genetically modified foods have antibiotic resistant genes in them. The imprecise technique used to transfer genes into a food has a very low success rate, so the scientists attach "marker genes" from bacteria that are resistant to antibiotics to help identify which cells have "taken" the new DNA. Scientists then douse the experimental GMO in antibiotics. If the GMO lives, they consider it a successful change to the DNA. The antibiotic-resistant marker genes commonly used are resistant to antibiotics used on humans and animals. Some scientists also fear that eating GM foods containing these antibiotic-resistant marker genes could transform the human gut bacteria to be antibiotic resistant.

Since so little research has been done on the safety of GM foods, it is not possible to know all of the risks. Now that they have been released into the environment, they may continue to pose risks to public health for centuries. In addition, genes in bacteria will transfer information to other genes as in the case with our gut bacteria. The long-term chronic exposure of our gut bacteria to antibiotic-resistant marker genes may continue to change the gut ecology long after we have discontinued consuming the GM food.

Polls have indicated that the U.S. population, given a choice, would not choose to eat GM foods. The biotech industry is using its financial might and political influence to keep from having to label foods that contain GMOs. Today, organic products often contain the No GMO label, but that may change. Most American consumers are unwittingly consuming GM foods, probably daily.

How do we avoid GMO foods? Thankfully, the overwhelming push back from the European Union, Africa, India and other countries has slowed the creation of many of the planned GM food crops. GMO foods on the market have been confined to the following foods: canola oil (rapeseed oil), chicory, radicchio, corn, cotton, papaya, potato, soybean, squash and tomato.

6
Home Is Where the Food Is

> *Most of us are creatures so comforted by habit, it can take something on the order of religion to invoke new, more conscious behaviors—however glad we may be afterward that we went to the trouble.*
> *– Barbara Kingsolver,* Animal, Vegetable, Miracle: A Year of Food Life

WHY BUY ORGANIC?

Organic food is good: good for the body; good for the environment; good for the farmer; and good for the farm worker. The Merriam-Webster English Dictionary defines organic in part as: 1) Organic Evolution: of, relating to, or derived from living organisms. 2) Organic Farming/Produce: of, relating to, yielding, or involving the use of food produced with the use of feed or fertilizer of plant or animal origin without employment of chemically formulated fertilizers, growth stimulants, antibiotics or pesticides.

The Environmental Protection Agency claims that conventional agriculture is responsible for 70 percent of the pollution to the country's rivers and streams caused by chemicals, erosion and toxic animal waste. If our food system can cause this much damage to our planet, imagine what it is doing to our bodies. Organic farming may be one of the last ways to keep both our ecosystems and our rural communities healthy and alive.

Small-scale organic farmers finance innovative research designed to reduce agricultural impact on the environment. They preserve biodiversity by collecting seeds and growing heirloom varieties of plants and rotate crops in the fields and plant cover crops to stop weeds, nutrient leaching and erosion. They naturally enrich the soil with manure and compost. Consumer demand is a powerful force for change. In 2007, the organic food industry grossed $23 billion worldwide and $10 billion in the U.S. alone. Every food category now has an organic alternative and many more non-food crops are grown organically each year. As consumers, we can help this trend continue by continuing to ask for and purchasing organically grown food, textiles, personal care and other items.

WHY BUY LOCAL?

Other than a fun and relaxing outing, why go to Farmers' Markets? Or, why participate in a Community Sponsored Agriculture (CSA) organization? Farmers' Markets and CSAs are win-win situations for the farmer or vendor and the consumer. The farmer can increase profits by selling directly to the consumer eliminating the middleman and creating a consistent revenue stream for the farm. The consumer profits from the availability of just picked, ripe produce fresh from the fields.

When you buy local, especially local organic, you are getting the best nature has to offer. Recognize that vegetables and fruits are seasonal, so the type of foods at a local farmers market will and should change. Shopping at local Farmers Markets or participating in a CSA helps you to stay in the rhythm of the season.

SHOPPING THE FARMERS' MARKET

When visiting a farmer's market, go early for the best selection unless you are a bargain shopper. Some vendors will drastically reduce their price near closing time. However, going late does risk a more limited availability because some vendors will sell out.

- Bring your own basket, cart or reusable bags with handles.
- Circulate first to see what is available before purchasing unless you have previously developed a relationship with a vendor.
- Dress comfortably.
- Enjoy the process of smelling and seeing the variety and choices at the stalls.

- Bring cash as most vendors will not accept credit cards or personal checks.
- Be adventurous and try something new. If you get something you have never tried before, use the Internet for recipes or preparation tips.
- Plan to return home soon after your shopping trip, or bring a cooler if it is hot outside. Leaving fresh produce in a hot car will compromise that "just picked" quality quickly.
- Shop often to ensure you are able to enjoy produce while it is fresh. Farmers' Markets are generally open on a set schedule allowing you to regularly purchase and eat produce at its peak during the seasons.

People erroneously assume that farmers' markets primarily offer organic produce. This is not always the case. Organic availability varies from vendor to vendor. Look for the organic label or ask the vendor. To display the approved organic seal the produce must contain at least 95 percent organically produced ingredients. The USDA's National Organic Program (NOP) regulates organic produce.

Farmers who produce certified organic foods do not use artificial fertilizers or pesticides. Additionally, organic foods are processed without artificial ingredients, genetically modified foods, preservatives or irradiation. We already know that organic produce does lower one's exposure to these toxins. If you can get organic locally, you are getting the best of both worlds.

There are serious local supporters called "locavores" who only eat foods grown within 100 miles of their homes. This new movement was nonexistent a few years ago, but has since become a part of mainstream vocabulary, particularly in urban cities such as San Francisco and New York. The most compelling reason many people choose to buy local is the carbon-emissions argument that buying local reduces the carbon-footprint. Yes, your organic avocado may have more frequent flyer miles than the most active cross-country salesperson. A typical potato has traveled 1,200 miles from Idaho; the typical carrot has traveled 1,600 miles from California, and a hamburger 600 miles from Colorado. On the surface, it seems obvious that local produce has a lower carbon footprint when compared to air freighted foods. But is reducing food miles necessarily good for the environment? Researchers have challenged the premise that more food miles automatically equate to greater fossil fuel consumption. According to the research, compelling evidence suggests that there are more inputs at stake than just travel miles and gas emissions.

Instead of measuring a product's carbon footprint through food miles alone, we should also include other energy-consuming aspects of production such as water use, harvesting techniques, fertilizer use, transportation and fuel use, as well as the disposal of packaging and storage procedures. Incorporating these measurements into the assessments, some scientists have reached shocking conclusions. Most notably, they found that all of the other factors could actually increase the "carbon footprint" even if the food was produced locally. These life-cycle measurements are causing environmentalists worldwide to rethink the logic of food miles.

So, yes, even buying local can also increase the carbon footprint. However, local farmers markets and CSAs are generally both better for you and better for the environment. There are other reasons for local purchasing. You are supporting a local businessperson who directly influences your local economy. When we collectively support local, especially organic, farmers, we also improve soil quality and fertility in our own regions while maintaining food diversity.

Conceptualize a hub-and-spoke system of food usage, with the hub being supporting local food producers and the spokes being the other sources for foods from supermarkets, markets, health food stores and specialty retailers to add to the diversity of what you eat.

HOW TO SHOP THE GROCERY STORE

One of my favorite activities is to give clients a guided tour of the grocery store. Unfortunately for many people, going to the grocery store can be a harrowing experience for many reasons: 1) Selecting the right foods can be overwhelming if you do not know what you are looking for. 2) Grocery stores are designed to encourage the consumer to buy more profitable foods; and in most cases profitable food equals nutrient-poor, low quality food. 3) Many people go to the store unprepared and even hungry, and what they end up putting in their cart can derail their healthy lifestyle goals. The reality is that the grocery store experience can be very exciting and fun once you know what you are doing.

IDENTIFY WHY YOU ARE SHOPPING

Food is the body's fuel and the nutrient content or lack thereof determines the quality of that fuel. Sadly, as Americans, we are often more concerned about what kind of gas to put in our cars than what kind of food we put in our bodies. Americans select foods based on taste, cost, convenience, appearance and shelf life. Oddly, none of these pertain to health, nutrient value or quality. If you are making all your food choices based on these criteria, you may be starving for nutrients and your health may be paying the price. It is not that you should ignore taste, cost, convenience, appearance and shelf life; these should be considerations. Nutritional content should be the primary factor when selecting foods, because nutrition is the real reason we need to eat.

Food, while it is providing us a sensory experience, is really fuel for the body to be used to make your cells, create your emotions, build muscle, fuel your mind and move your body. All of these processes need the nutrients in food to be able to perform optimally. Nutrients are the catalysts and building blocks of the body.

So where do you go once you decide to focus on a food's nutritional value? There are ways to navigate the grocery store to come out with the most nutritious food available, and the following principles should help to guide you along your way.

Be Prepared

The number one rule of grocery shopping is to never go to the store hungry. With hunger gnawing at your stomach, you are more likely to make poor choices regardless of your intention before getting there.

Go to the store prepared with a list. Just like anything else we do, preparation is required and often the deciding factor in success. Keep a note pad on the refrigerator or in the kitchen to keep track of when you run out or get low on staple items. Write down what you need as you run out. Then, go through your refrigerator and pantry noting on your list what items you need before embarking on your shopping trip.

Plan your meals before making your list and shopping. If you use recipes when cooking, look at the recipes that you intend to make and add the ingredients to your shopping list. The Cleanse Program provides a lot of recipes from which to create your shopping list. Also, you have a list of foods allowed on The Cleanse Program, so you can even use those foods to make your own recipes.

Shop the Perimeter

Most grocery stores are designed with the non-perishables along the interior sections of the store. The foods with the highest nutrient content are along the perimeter. The more you shop along the perimeter, the better. Vegetables, fruits and lean cuts of protein found along the perimeter should be the bulk of your shopping trip, with quick excursions to the center for key non-perishable items such as legumes and whole grains.

Fresh is Best, Frozen is Better, Canned in a Crunch

Start with the freshest ingredients: fresh fruits and vegetables. When buying vegetables, local organic produce is the best option. Once fresh fruits and vegetables are picked, they start to lose their nutrient content. Most organic produce will travel thousands of miles before making it to your grocery cart. So when you buy fresh, be aware that you will want to eat these foods soon to have the best taste and nutrient content.

Local, organic produce is the best produce choice. If you have access to organic, don't just pass it up because you assume it is too expensive. Sometimes organic food is actually less expensive than traditionally grown food, especially when it is on sale. Be sure to compare prices and choose the best value, which may in fact be organic.

Organic, non-local produce is your next best bet. Organic does have better food value and will reduce your exposure to pesticides, herbicides and other toxins. Remember, conventionally grown produce is exposed to insecticides, herbicides and poor soil quality. The result is conventionally grown food is tainted with chemicals that often cannot be washed off. Organic farmers use natural predators, crop rotation and natural fertilizers to enable the crops to grow. Now, if organic produce is hard to find, it is better to eat conventionally grown produce than no produce at all.

It is always a good idea to have a stash of flash frozen vegetables in the freezer in a pinch. As a last result, canned vegetables are also good to have on hand. However, canned vegetables are the least nutritious options. Canned vegetables lose some of their vitamin C content during the canning process.

Free-Range Beef and Fowl

Organic, free-range meats and poultry are always the best choice. Organic meats are by definition free from antibiotics and hormones. "Free-range" implies that the animal was raised in its natural environment and not in feedlots. However, with free-range, be sure to check your sources and make sure this is an honest claim. If you do not have access to organic, free-range meat and poultry, select the leanest cuts as most of the toxins from hormones and antibiotics will settle in the meat's fatty tissue. If you buy conventional poultry, do not eat the skin as it contains the highest concentration of toxins.

Remember the label "Natural" does not have any teeth behind it, meaning that there are no regulations defining what makes something natural. So do not be duped by the hype. Look for other labeling such as "free from pesticides, hormones and herbicides."

Just as organic, local produce is your best choice, supporting local, organic free-range meat and poultry producers are also your ideal source. The Slow Foods' Web site is an excellent resource for finding local, sustainable farmers and ranchers in your area. (www.SlowFoods.com)

WILD-CAUGHT FISH VS. FARM-RAISED FISH

It is no secret that fish can contain toxins such as mercury and PCBs. Much like feedlots, farm-raised fish are caged in pens inside the ocean without the ability to swim or move freely. Farm-raised fish are prone to disease, and are therefore fed antibiotics. Farm-raised fish often have higher levels of mercury. For instance, wild salmon become pink by eating krill, which contains a carotenoid called astaxanthin. Farmed salmon are naturally grayish but are given artificial colorings to make them more appealing to the consumer. Obviously, we want our food to look as it does in nature. The chemicals used to convert the gray, farm-raised salmon to a "natural" pink are canthaxanthin and astaxanthin. Some farm-raised salmon fillets are also dyed with food dye to match the wild-caught coloring. Farm-raised salmon contain lower amounts of the valuable omega-3 fat. Always choose fresh, ocean-caught Alaskan salmon, fresh sardines or anchovies over farm-raised fish.

A Note About Dairy

As you know, dairy is not on The Cleanse Program, but for future reference, there are some guidelines to follow when buying dairy. Free-range, organic dairy products are the best option. Conventional dairy cows are one of the most heavily drugged and mistreated of all farm animals. Conventionally farmed dairy cows are given bovine growth hormone (rBST) to keep the cows steadily producing milk. The use of rBST has diminished in the last few years due to consumer outcry, but some commercial producers still use it. Studies show that ingesting bovine growth hormone significantly increases the levels of the human growth hormone factor IGF-1, which is associated with elevated levels of insulin, increased growth hormones and can also lead to increased cell production. Dairy cows live in crowded conditions that breed disease and therefore require high levels of antibiotics. Consequently, these antibiotics end up in the milk, cheese and yogurt produced by the conventional dairy and into the bodies of the humans who ingest these products.

Dairy is not the best source of calcium, as you have already learned. The following vegetables have the same amount of calcium as a glass of milk:

- 1½ cups of cooked kale
- 2¾ cups of cooked broccoli
- 8 cups of cooked spinach

Shop the Interior of the Store Sparingly

The majority of the sales floor of a grocery store is devoted to processed foods. This is where the most profits are made and the least nutritious foods are shelved. Processed foods are among the most nutritionally devoid foods. The best rule of thumb is the more packaging and marketing behind the product, the less healthy it is for you. Save the money that you would normally spend on pricey and unhealthy items such as potato chips, cookies, ice cream, frozen pizzas and pasta casseroles and spend it on some fresh vegetables or meat instead.

Label Lunacy

With the release of the latest Food Pyramid, created by the U.S. Department of Agriculture, the confusion around food value has become even more contentious with processed foods stating erroneous labels such as "made with whole grains," or a "good source of vitamins and minerals." For instance, a "good source of vitamins" as outlined by the USDA means that one serving of a food contains 10 to 19 percent of the daily required nutrients.

Whole Grains

One of the most troubling food label slide of hands is what constitutes "whole grain." Whole grains are very easy to spot. The only real whole grain is the seed or kernel as it comes from the plant without any processing. You know you have never seen amber waves of toast as you ride down the roadway! Whole grains are just how they are found in nature—brown rice, whole oat groat, barley, millet, brown rice and quinoa. Once a grain has been crushed, milled, flaked or baked, it has been altered and its nutrient value compromised. Whole wheat bread "made with whole grain" is not a whole grain. It may contain some whole grain particles, but the majority of the grain has been milled into flour that increases the speed in which it is digested and made into sugar by the body. When looking for whole grains, look for grain in its natural state. Note: Gluten-containing grains such as wheat, rye, barley and spelt are not on The Cleanse Program nor are any processed grain foods.

Whole Foods = Healthy Body

Upgrading your shopping savvy at the grocery store is an essential step to creating a healthier body. Whole foods contain the highest nutrient content, and therefore lead a healthier body. Health is our most important possession. Just like your car, it deserves high quality fuel. Shop the perimeter of the supermarket and only go to the center for specific, pre-planned items (e.g., real whole grains, nuts, bottled water and toiletries). Avoid the overwhelming marketing aimed at your pocketbook and not at your health.

7
It Takes Guts

> *The part can never be well unless the whole is well.*
> *– Plato*

LINDA JACKSON, TESTIMONIAL

I started The Cleanse Program primarily to address my acid-reflux and general digestive health. Weight loss was a concern, but it was secondary to my newly acquired digestive discomfort.

After participating in the three-week program, I no longer experience bloating after a meal or during the day. I also have a new, general feeling of health, and I no longer feel heavy in my stomach during the day.

During the entire program I slept like a baby! It was amazing. I would get up in the morning feeling totally refreshed! My newfound sleep made me realize how much food affects sleep patterns.

Prior to starting the three-week cleanse program, I was really worried about being able to cope with cooking and meal planning. I eat out frequently and travel often. I was shocked by how simple it is to eat out and cook without completely changing my routine! I now have some new favorite meals and have discovered new foods that I really enjoy. I even crave some of the components of The Cleanse Program such as the water and juice combination.

I feel much better after The Cleanse Program, and I have slept better than I have in years. By combining The Cleanse Program with the IgG-food sensitivity blood test, my acid-reflux has disappeared. To echo the words of my pulmonologist—*hallelujah*! Neither my doctor nor I had any idea my persistent cough had anything to do with food.

After reintroducing foods, I found that soy seemed to be a culprit in my cough and reflux. I am careful now about consuming the foods I now know my body does not respond well to, but I do still enjoy the occasional ice cream or glass of wine in the evening. The difference is that now I know how much I can eat and how often before I experience negative symptoms.

I have continued the morning Cleanse Meal Replacement. I even take the ingredients with me when I travel. I have also continued drinking water with juice. I feel so empowered knowing that I can change my eating habits and literally change my life.

Our bodies have several "inputs"—ways in which it receives and processes information. One input is from the environment—what the body is exposed to both internally and externally. Another input is what the body uses to operate day-to-day as raw materials. Environment (exposures) and raw materials (nutrients) make up the information and nourishment that our body uses to affect our day-to-day lives.

Example: In the hotter climates of the U.S., people endure incredibly hot summers. Water rationing and reductions are an annual way of life. So watering the lawn becomes a luxury. While homeowners are not able to water the lawn, they must be sure to water the foundation (building blocks) of the house in order to prevent cracking. Because the ground is made of clay (heredity), it will shrink and form large cracks in its surface. When dry, the ground pulls away from the foundation of the house and can create an unstable surface for the house. The house then shifts causing cracks in the interior walls. If, however, homeowners keep the foundation moist (environment stable and ideal), the foundation remains intact. If homeowners do not water the foundation, the house will crack.

To take this analogy further, let us look at what you would do if you noticed your house cracking. If you had a house where the foundation was suddenly cracking, you would ask yourself two major questions: 1) Is there an environmental reason or exposure that is causing damage to occur to the structure of the house? (In this case, a drought.) 2) Is there something the structure of the house requires that it is not getting? (In this case, water). The solution is a simple, two-pronged approach.

Just as in the example of the house, in order to understand what has initiated an imbalance in the body and determine the cause of the biochemical malfunctions, we must ask ourselves these same two questions: What environmental exposures could be at play and what is missing?

For example, let's say Sally has gas and bloating with discomfort after eating. In the U.S., Sally would most likely see a doctor and probably get diagnosed (symptom labeling) with IBS and get an anti-spasmodic medication to stop the symptoms (alarms from the body). The drug may suppress (treat) Sally's symptoms, but the cause of the illness is by no means gone.

Another perspective: Sally has digestive discomfort after eating (exposure to environment). What could be the things leading to the symptoms? It could be what she ate, or how fast she ate it. It could also be that her body is lacking some nutrient(s) that aids in digestion. The diagnosis of IBS is merely a label. The examination of all the possible factors influencing the bloating, gas and discomfort is the basis for removing the symptoms (traditionally referred to as a diagnosis) that is essential in healing the disease as opposed to treating the symptoms.

Once these questions have been answered, it is then possible to systematically go through a process of taking care of the factors contributing to the symptom and the missing factors that may be causing the symptoms. You may have heard the saying, "All health relies on the health of the gut." This is a true claim. Seventy-five percent of the immune system resides in the gut; we assimilate nutrients from the gut to run, repair and rebuild our bodies. To be healthy, the gut must be healthy. The Cleanse Program is designed to start bringing a high degree of health back to the gut.

FIVE R'S TO HEALING THE GUT

Gut healing involves four components: remove, re-inoculate, replace and repair.

- Remove: Eliminate anything that may be in the body or diet that contributes to poor health. This can include foods, food additives, unwanted bacteria, fungi, parasites, metals and environmental toxins such as pesticides.
- Re-inoculate: Implement a regimen of probiotic supplements containing friendly flora. These bacteria repel harmful microbes and have anti-tumor effects. Gut flora is easily disrupted by use of antibiotics and the stress of contemporary living.
- Replace: Support the body's biochemical functions by replacing non-nutritive foods with highly dense foods and supplements.
- Repair: Quickly regenerate and heal the body with nutritional support.
- Rebalance: Lifestyle choices such as sleep, exercise and stress can all affect the GI tract.

The first step in The Cleanse Program is to remove anything that may be in your environment that is causing negative symptoms. This may include foods, chemicals, as well as toxic thoughts and relationships. When the body is alarmed by foods, it responds much like it responds to a virus or bacterial infection by launching a war between the immune system cells, the food and your body tissues. For a complete discussion about immune responses to foods, refer back to chapter three: When "Healthy" Food Hurts.

The eight most common food allergens that elicit an immune system response in the body along with some toxins that have become a ubiquitous part of our eating culture are the first items removed from your diet on The Cleanse Program. Many of the foods on the "do not eat" list are common derivatives used in the manufacturing process of processed foods. Before the advent of the food processing industry, most of the foods we ate were whole or minimally processed. Since World War II, much of the supermarket is comprised of foods made from six main ingredients: wheat, corn, soy, egg, yeast and dairy. You may be surprised to learn that you probably eat these same six ingredients at every meal and most of your calories consist of calories made up of these six foods.

A HOLISTIC APPROACH TO WELL-BEING: STARTING WITH THE GUT

In Western medicine, the digestive tract takes a back seat to the blood, heart and circulatory system as the primary tool for diagnostics and healing. In the West, little attention is paid to the foods we eat and the balance of our digestive system. Conversely, according to Ayurveda, the medical system started in India, and Chinese medicine (both over 5000 years old), digestion is the cornerstone of well-being and health. Both systems traditionally use the digestive organs as a tool for diagnoses. For example, in both systems, the tongue is used to determine digestive strength and health of the body. Your bowel movement frequency and consistency is also an important discussion determining absorption of nutrients.

While studying the basic tenets of Ayurvedic medicine, meditation and yoga in India, I was encouraged to learn that a good portion of the Ayurvedic intake process a doctor goes through is regarding food, lifestyle and digestion. This experience only strengthened my resolve to delve deeper into the digestive process as a tool to help the body recover.

We cannot ignore the single-most important environmental input (food) and function in the body (digestion) and assume to be able to stay well and heal our bodies. Food and digestion are the two the most important environmental inputs.

CLEANSING TO OPTIMIZE YOUR HORMONES

The Cleanse Program will have several positive effects on your body. First, and foremost, this program will assist in bringing balance to the digestive system. There are a lot of people running around with sluggish digestion, IBS symptoms and other digestive complaints who believe they are "normal." However, any type of negative digestive symptom is anything but a "normal" state. People with digestive ailments may be in the majority, but that does not mean their bodies are functioning normally. Normal digestive function is eating with no painful side effects: heartburn, reflux, GERD, stomachache, bloating, gas, cramping, hemorrhoids, constipation or diarrhea.

All this digestive discomfort affects our well-being, our hormones and endocrine system. For example, when the body has utilized the estrogen it has produced at the cellular level, the estrogen is moved to the liver to be detoxified. Once the estrogen is detoxified through chemical reactions, it is sent to the intestines in the bile to be mixed with fiber to be excreted. If your diet does not have enough fiber to absorb and bind up the estrogen, you will reabsorb the estrogen in the intestinal lining causing it to continue to re-circulate in the blood. This alone can lead to elevated estrogen, weight gain from estrogen dominance and heightened hormonal imbalances. So, what we eat, and how we digest has significant impact on our hormones.

First, the diet must consist of fiber in order for the body to operate at optimal levels. Dietary fiber is generally considered indigestible to humans and is broadly classified as water-soluble and water-insoluble fibers.

Benefits of fiber:

- Water-insoluble fibers bind or attract water making them very viscous, which adds bulk to the stool. This bulking helps maintain normal bowel function by acting as a scouring agent in the bowel.
- Water-soluble fibers actually dissolve in water and are used as a food source by the bacteria in the intestines.
- Dietary fiber is important to human health and nutrition because of its role in regulating blood sugar (glucose) by slowing the speed in which carbohydrates are broken down and digested, thereby causing a slower rise in blood sugar and

reducing the inflammatory response to food.

- Fiber assists in cholesterol absorption by binding to cholesterol in the digestive tract and pulling it out of the body.
- Fiber helps with detoxification and elimination by binding with toxins, food additives and hormones such as estrogen and cortisol.
- Fiber will improve satiety after eating.

The best sources of dietary fiber:

- High-fiber vegetables include many of the green leafy vegetables such as kale, collard greens, chard, arugula and even some lettuces.
- Fibrous fruits such as apple, papaya, berries and pears.
- Tree nuts are a great source of dietary fiber and good fats.
- Whole-grain sources of fiber include quinoa, millet, amaranth and brown rice.
- Legumes include beans such as peas, lentils, black, field peas and chickpeas.

Quick sources of supplemental fiber include ground flax seed (freshly ground to preserve the oils present in the seeds), and psyllium husk supplements, chopped nuts, and/or freeze-dried vegetable fiber. These fibers can be sprinkled over foods—cooked vegetables, salads and mixed in protein shakes or water. As you might have guessed, the great forms of fiber mentioned above are in rich supply on The Cleanse Program.

The typical American has an intake of fiber between five and 10gm per day. A Paleolithic period man ate an average of 100gm of fiber daily! Wow, how our diet has worsened. The current USDA recommended intake is 30gm–50gm per day. Having this much natural fiber, keeps the digestive system moving and helps the body excrete metabolized hormones and toxins. While on The Cleanse Program, you will need to increase your water intake as you increase the fiber intake to avoid constipation due to the water-binding/bulking effects of water-insoluble fibers.

Fiber is not the only change that we will be making to your diet. Increasing and balancing good fats can also optimize your body functions. Inflammation, the body's most primitive weapon against infection and injury, may be at the root of some of the deadliest diseases including heart disease, diabetes, cancer and Alzheimer's. What we eat has a direct impact on our level of inflammation—particularly the fats we eat.

Inflammation

So what does fat have to do with inflammation? It has everything to do with it. Here's how the inflammatory cycle can spin out of control. Under normal circumstances, inflammation is an immune reaction that helps the body heal when injured. Heat, swelling and soreness on a cut or bruise are all part of the inflammation process. However, inflammation can become chronic or prolonged with deleterious effects on the body.

Medical researchers discovered long ago that certain diseases such as lupus, Graves' and fibromyalgia emerge when the immune system kicks into overdrive without turning off. This same process occurs in cardiovascular disease. Until the early 1990s, medical experts believed that heart disease, specifically atherosclerosis (hardening of the arteries), resulted when sticky plaque stuck to smooth artery walls causing the narrowing of the artery. If you had a heart attack, it was from a blood clot plugging the artery. As it turns out, however, heart disease is more complex than that. Arteries absorb the LDL cholesterol from the bloodstream between the tissue layers of the arteries. This creates a kind of blister or bubble as opposed to the LDL cholesterol sticking to the artery wall. The body may then trigger an inflammatory response to the blister on the wall of the artery constricting blood flow to the heart. Disaster finally strikes when the blister (plaque) bursts and the inflammatory debris clogs the artery.

Guess what? Your fat cells are also increasing your level of inflammation. Our fat cells are little power stations producing inflammation-boosting proteins called cytokines. The more body fat a person has, the more inflammation he or she will have. Over time, the constant increase in cytokines hampers the body's ability to monitor insulin production (insulin manages blood sugar) and the inflammation goes unchecked and you are now at risk for diabetes and cardiovascular disease and many other diseases.

Chronic inflammation also causes oxidative stress or over production of free radicals (rusting) on the cells that may trigger cellular mutations (e.g., cancer).

Inflammation has been implicated in Alzheimer's. Although the mechanism is not fully understood, neurologists believe the brain's immune cells attack the plaquing in the brain that signals Alzheimer's. The ensuing skirmish creates inflammation that may spur progression of the disease.

Most foods either fuel the fires of inflammation or help extinguish them. Fat is at the center of the issue. The goal is to eat a good balance of anti-inflammatory fats such as the omega-3s found in fish and the omega-9s found in olive oil or avocado and a limited amount of the inflammatory fats such as the omega-6 oils found in safflower, sunflower and canola. The typical American diet of processed foods, fast foods and restaurant foods is full of pro-inflammatory omega-6 fats like corn and soy oils.

The two key omega-3 fatty acids are eicosapentaenoic (EPA) and docosahexaenoic (DHA). These are potent anti-inflammatory fats that are hard to obtain in our diet. Good sources are fatty fish such as mackerel, salmon, trout, sardines and tuna. Omega-3 fats can also be obtained from seeds such as flax, hemp and walnuts.

You do need to watch out for toxins in fish, especially if you are pregnant or hoping to become pregnant. You should avoid tuna, shark, king mackerel, swordfish and tilefish, as these harbor potentially dangerous levels of mercury, which can be damaging to developing fetuses and nursing children. Fish oil supplements may be the better option since it is challenging to find fresh, mercury-free fish. Fish oil supplements are not required on The Cleanse Program, but may be helpful. I consider supplemental high quality fish oil mandatory for maintaining long-term health for everyone. You can purchase high quality fish oil at www.CleanseTheBook.com.

Although there are omega-3 options for vegetarians, they are not perfect. The body can make its own EPA and DHA from the omega-3 fat found in plant sources such as flaxseed and walnuts. But the body's mechanism for converting plant-based omega-3s is not particularly effective. The body must go through a rather taxing and arduous process to convert alpha-linolenic acid to the longer chain EPA and DHA fatty acids found in fish oils. Flax oil is good but not quite equal to fish oils.

Now that you know what you will be increasing on The Cleanse Program, let's look at what you be removing or decreasing. Remove trans-fats from your diet. Period! There is nothing positive about trans-fats. Trans-fats are the worst offenders because they up-regulate inflammation. The worst culprits are vegetable shortenings, margarines and processed foods.

Balancing fat intake will have a significant affect on inflammation and will affect your hormones, specifically the hormone signaling molecules such as cytokines. When these molecules become balanced, the body's hormone messages also become balanced, reducing symptoms such as blood sugar highs and lows as well as weight (fat) gain around the belly.

Protein intake plays an important role in stabilizing hormones. Proteins provide 22 amino acids required by the human body, most importantly the eight essential amino acids (those that cannot be made by the body). Amino acids are the end result of protein digestion and are the building blocks of the body. Proteins comprise the body's cells, function as enzymes and hormones, and act as transport carriers in membranes.

Protein plays a role in food regulation, satiety and functions distinct from the provision of energy. The daily intake of protein in healthy amounts and lowering the amount of processed and non-nutritive carbohydrates will stabilize blood levels of glucose and insulin. Proper levels of protein intake reduce your insulin response after you eat, which is a good thing. Lower insulin levels equals reduced risk for diabetes and weight gain. Caveat: too much protein at meals is counter-productive and can lead to an acidic body, and even can cause an over-production of insulin in response to the large meal.

Acid Alkaline Balance

Our western diet is full of grains and shelf-stable food products devoid of essential nutritional components that increase the acid load in our bodies. Our Standard American Diet (SAD) is rotting our bodies like a tooth in a can of cola. Cola, through its acid content, will rot a human tooth in a matter of days. Processed, sugar-laden foods do the same thing to our body and bones.

On the other hand, diets high in fruits and vegetables are associated with a greater degree of alkalinity. Alkaline-forming foods are primarily vegetables and fruits, while acid-forming foods are derived from cheese, meat, fish and grain products (i.e., your packaged foods).

Over time, ingestion of a high dietary acid load can progress to a chronic, low-grade level of over-acidity. A chronic acidic load can cause a number of health conditions such as osteoporosis, kidney disease and muscle wasting.

In order to maintain acid-alkaline balance throughout the various body systems, one system may be required to support another. For example, the bones contain minerals that alkalize such as calcium and magnesium. The minerals are released from the bones to balance or buffer (such as Alkaseltzer) an overly acidic dietary load in the event of inadequate buffering capacity in the blood. Repeated borrowing of the body's alkaline reserve in response to a consistent increased (dietary) acid load can be potentially detrimental.

Conversely, changing your alkalinity can positively influence bone metabolism. A diet favoring balanced acid and alkalinity increases calcium absorption. Furthermore, studies have demonstrated a positive link between a high intake of alkali-rich fruits and vegetables with preservation of bone mineral density.

Although it is not common, blood pH levels can shift to the side of excessive acidity or alkalinity, in both cases several clinical symptoms will appear. Acidosis can lead to symptoms of lethargy, while alkalosis can lead to cramps, muscle spasms, irritability and hyper-excitability.

This concept of acid-alkaline balance is becoming more and more embraced within the medical community. Naturopathic medicine has used the acid-alkaline balance as a model to explain the foundation of many diseases. Allopathic medicine has examined pH in specific organ systems such as the kidney to control the formation of stones and the elimination of toxins.

On The Cleanse Program, we will be consuming a lot of natural fiber, good fats, enough but not too much protein, and balancing the acidity of the body with an abundance of vegetables and fruits. Just doing these few things alone often can reverse several symptoms you may be dealing with such as lethargy, sluggish digestion, sleep disturbances and digestive upset.

8
Digestion: A User's Guide

> *Now good digestion waits on appetite,*
> *and health on both! – William Shakespeare*

Knowledge is power, and since there is a high probability that many of us were daydreaming in high school health class or checking out the backs of our eyelids in biology, this chapter will serve as a useful refresher on just how the digestive system should function. If the complex action of digestion is a fine-tuned, well running machine, and we are feeding it high-quality fuel, we can slow the aging and disease forming process. Take this opportunity to reacquaint yourself with the journey food takes through your body.

The human digestive system is a complex series of organs and glands that help turn food into fuel and repair molecules. In order to use the food we eat, our body has to break the food down into smaller molecules that it can process; it also has to trash the leftover waste. Good health relies on healthy digestion.

The stomach and intestines are the main digestive organs. These tube-like organs contain the food as it makes its way through the body. The digestive system is essentially a long, twisting tube that runs from the mouth to the anus. The digestive system produces and stores digestive chemicals required to breakdown the food. The digestive tract is designed to keep its contents separate from the other organs until the nutrients can be extracted and sent to the bloodstream.

THE DIGESTIVE PROCESS

Digestion starts in the mouth, which is, of course, the first part of the gastrointestinal tract. The mouth is comprised of the lips, cheeks, tongue, palate and teeth. It receives secretions from the salivary glands, which help to start the digestion process. Our mouths perform four main functions: mastication (chewing), early digestion of carbohydrates, breathing and speech.

The mouth breaks food into small particles by mastication with the teeth and mixing food with saliva. The chewing process forms what is called a bolus (imagine a ball of food mixed together), and allows swallowing and tasting of foods. The mouth is a passageway to the esophagus down to the stomach. The mouth is also a passageway between the pharynx (the cavity connecting the nose, mouth and larynx) and the outside of the body. This allows us to breath both through the nose and the mouth.

In the mouth, we produce saliva to assist in the creation of the bolus. Saliva contains amylase, a digestive enzyme responsible for initiating the process of breaking down carbohydrates. Some experts also believe that salivary amylase may have agonistic effects on pancreatic output of insulin, meaning that the secretion of amylase triggers the pancreas to secrete insulin to respond to the carbohydrate (sugars) tasted in the mouth. So even in the mouth, the digestive process is in high gear!

STOMACH

The stomach is a sack-like shaped organ located between the esophagus and the intestines. The stomach changes size and shape according to the position of the body and the amount of food inside it. The average stomach is about 12-inches long and is six-inches wide at its widest point. The stomach's capacity is about one quart in an adult. The stomach is composed of five layers. The innermost layer is called the mucosa. Stomach acid and digestive juices are made in the mucosa layer; the mucosa layer is covered in mucus to protect the other layers from hydrochloric acid produced in the mucosal layer. The next four layers are layers of muscle that moves with the action of peristalsis and mixes the stomach contents just like a squeeze bottle. These muscles are what you feel when your stomach is turning or growling.

Food enters the stomach from the esophagus. The valve, or door between the stomach and the esophagus, is called the cardiac sphincter. The cardiac sphincter prevents food from passing back to the esophagus. The cardiac sphincter is located next to the heart (the reason for its name). Its proximity to the heart is why many people who suffer from heartburn or GERD feel as though they may be having a heart attack at times because the pain and burning can be similar in both situations.

Once the food enters the stomach, gastric juices are used to deconstruct the food. Gastric juice is a strong acidic liquid with a pH of one to three in humans. The hormone gastrin is released into the bloodstream when protein peptides are detected in the stomach. This causes gastric glands in mucosa to secrete gastric juice. Gastric juices are collectively hydrochloric acid and the digestive enzymes pepsin, protease and DPP IV. All of these are responsible for breaking down proteins in all foods in the stomach.

One of the most common symptoms of a poorly functioning stomach is heartburn or reflux (GERD). The unfortunate truth is the mainstream treatment for heartburn and reflex often mask the real issue of reduced hydrochloric acid and pepsin production. Low production of pepsin and hydrochloric acid can actually increase the sensation of GERD due to foods, particularly protein, sitting in the stomach waiting for the pH to get low enough to start the digestive process thereby causing gastric juices to bubble past the cardiac sphincter. The amount of acid in the stomach of a GERD sufferer is usually in normal levels.

Some substances, alcohol and fructose in particular, are absorbed directly through the muscle lining of the stomach for a straight shot to the liver.

The problem derives from the acid being in the wrong location. Instead of staying in the stomach, it moves into the esophagus from the slowing of gastric emptying because of low acid or overeating. While heartburn caused by acid reflux in the esophagus is the most common symptom of GERD, it is not the only effect on the body. Another important condition that may be caused by, or worsened by, acid reflux is asthma. In recent studies, GERD was found to cause or exacerbate asthma, but that asthma and asthma medications may in turn cause or aggravate GERD. Sufferers may also experience hoarseness caused by irritation from acid reflux around the vocal cords or a chronic cough and sore throat. While stress can worsen heartburn, it is rare for it to be the sole cause of heartburn.

While on The Cleanse Program, you may experience a reduction or even a complete remission of GERD symptoms. Heartburn can be corrected through a change in diet, maintaining proper portion control and taking digestive enzymes with betaine HCL and pepsin. If GERD is a chronic symptom for you, it is important to keep a food log or diary to discover the foods that trigger your heartburn. In some cases of GERD, spicy foods, carbonation, acidic foods and rich foods may increase symptoms.

Nearly 60 million American adults suffer from heartburn at least once a month. Chronic heartburn can be a symptom of one or more serious conditions including Barrett's esophagus, erosive esophagitis, eosinophilic esophagitis (caused by food allergies) and even esophageal cancer. If you continue to experience reoccurring GERD even after trying dietary changes, you should seek help from a health care practitioner to rule out other causes and concerns.

SMALL INTESTINES

The lower end of the stomach empties into the duodenum. The duodenum is the first section of the small intestine. The pyloric sphincter separates the stomach from the duodenum.

In the small intestine, after being in the stomach, food enters the duodenum, the first part of the small intestine. It then enters the jejunum and then the ileum, which is the final part of the small intestine. In the small intestine, bile that is produced in the liver and stored in the gall bladder along with pancreatic enzymes and other digestive enzymes produced by the inner wall of the small intestine help in the breakdown of food.

The enzymes in the small intestine convert the acidic chyme in the stomach to an alkaline substance and assist in further deconstructing the foods into their smallest component parts such as amino acids, fatty acids, carbohydrates and fiber. The duodenum is the first section of the small intestine and is connected to the stomach. The duodenum initiates the breakdown of food before moving it into the jejunum. The jejunum absorbs most of the nutrients into the bloodstream. The next stop on the journey is the ileum where vitamin B12, bile salts and the final processing of proteins and carbohydrates occur. The ileum is the last portion of the small intestine and connects to the large intestine.

Unlike the outer walls of the small intestine, the inner walls are made up of two types of wrinkles and folds called plicae circulares and rugae. The plicae circulares are a fixed feature of the small intestinal walls, while the rugae allow extra tissue for the small intestine to distend and contract as needed. The plicae circulares have two finger-like projections called villi (a Latin word meaning "shaggy hair") and microvilli. The microvilli cover the villi like a velvet coating. These two kinds of fine, frond-like protrusions work together to maximize the small intestine surface for ultra-efficient nutrient absorption. Each villus is the home of lacteal lymphatic capillaries that absorb fats and circulatory capillaries, which are close to the surface to absorb other nutrients.

The villi are often subject to damage due to poor diet, pathogen infection and food allergies and sensitivities. It is in the small intestine where damage occurs causing mal-absorption and other bodily problems.

LARGE INTESTINES

After food passes through the small intestine, it travels into the large intestine. The large intestine is four to five feet long. In the large intestine, some of the water and electrolytes—cell salts (chemicals such as sodium and potassium)—are removed from the food.

The first part of the large intestine is called the cecum (the appendix is connected to the cecum). Food then is pushed by peristalsis upward in the ascending colon. The food travels across the abdomen in the transverse colon, goes back down the other side of the body in the descending colon, and then through the sigmoid colon at the end. The large intestines have a mucosal barrier that protects it from pathogens attaching to the intestinal wall. Solid waste is then stored in the rectum until it is excreted via the anus.

Over three to seven pounds of bacteria live and colonize in both the small and large intestines. Bacteria belongs in our intestines—without it, we would die. We have a symbiotic relationship with intestinal bacteria; we cannot exist without the bacteria, much like Paris Hilton and the paparazzi. These bacteria also create many of the vitamins required by the body such as vitamin K and biotin.

Many microbes such as the bacteria bifidobacterium, lactobacillus acidophilus, escherichia coli and klebsiella inhabit the large intestine and assist in the digestion process. Bifidobacteria are also abundant and are often described as "friendly bacteria." These little guys are also very sensitive to bodily stress and the acid/alkaline balance in the body. So, high stress can also cause a deathblow to the gut bacteria.

In the large intestine, the good bacteria causes a fermenting action on the fiber from our diet to make short-chain fatty acids that serve as its food source. A low fiber diet will actually cause a famine in the gut and destroy the "good guy" bacteria, essentially starving it to death. A diet low in fiber will also give pathenogenic (bad guys such as candida and clostridium difficle) a continuous food source of sugars allowing them to thrive and kill the good guys. A poor diet is like providing funding to the intestinal drug lords.

Other bacterial products include gas, which is a mixture of nitrogen and carbon dioxide, methane and hydrogen sulphide all of which is produced by bacterial fermentation of undigested starch. When your digestion is not working well, or you have too little good bacteria, foods pass through the intestines undigested leaving starches intact to feed intestinal yeast and bad bacteria all of which can create gas and bloating.

Good gut bacteria are also involved in the production of cross-reactive antibodies. These are antibodies produced by the immune system against the normal flora that are also effective against related pathogens, thereby preventing infection or invasion. The most prevalent bacteria in the large intestines are the bacteroides. When bacteroides overgrow, they can produce symptoms of colitis and colon cancer.

The bacteria in our bodies are there to help us live. Much like the small ground plants, insects and small animals assist the trees in the forest, the digestive tract is an ecosystem that can be balanced or unbalanced based on environmental influences. Your diet either tip that balance toward a healthy forest or one that has been leveled for bad bacteria and yeast condos. It is up to you.

PANCREAS

The pancreas is an organ in the digestive and endocrine system. It is both an endocrine gland producing several important hormones, including insulin, glucagon and somatostatin, as well as an exocrine gland, secreting pancreatic juice containing digestive enzymes such as lipase and amylase into the small intestine. These enzymes assist in the further breakdown of the carbohydrates, protein and fat in the chyme.

The part of the pancreas involved in endocrine function is comprised of a group of cells called the islets of Langerhans. These cells are a compact collection of endocrine cells arranged in clusters and cords and are crisscrossed by a dense network of blood stream capillaries. These are the cells responsible for producing insulin, somatostatin and glucagon. Insulin has two main jobs: 1) move sugar into the body cells for burning, or 2) store sugar as fat for later use. Somatasostatin suppresses other hormone activities such as the repair activities of growth hormone and slowing the secretions of the pancreas. Glucagon's function is to cause the liver to release stored glucose from its cells into the blood. Glucagon is also used in the production of glucose by the liver out of building blocks obtained from other nutrients found in the body (e.g., protein). During fasting, the body uses glucagon as a signal to scavenge protein from muscles to be converted in the liver to glucose through the process of gluconeogenesis.

In contrast to the endocrine function of the pancreas, which secretes hormones into the blood, the exocrine activities of the pancreas produces digestive enzymes and an alkaline fluid (referred to as pancreatic juice), and secretes them into the small intestine. The hormones secretin and cholecystokinin signal this process. Digestive enzymes include trypsin, chymotrypsin, pancreatic lipase and pancreatic amylase.

The pancreas is vital to our survival. How we eat, and what we eat has a profound influence on the function and vitality of the pancreas. So, the next time you feel the urge to grab a sugary soft drink, remember your pancreas is going to run a marathon to produce enough insulin to handle all that sugar.

GALL BLADDER

The gallbladder is a small, pear-shaped, muscular sack that acts as a storage tank for bile. Bile is made in the liver. Bile is secreted through tiny ducts or canals to the duodenum (small intestine) and to the gallbladder. The gallbladder stores the bile to have it available in larger quantities for secretion when a meal is eaten. The ingestion of food, especially fats, causes the release of a hormone called cholecystokinin (CCK), which signals the bile to enter the small intestine. It also signals the contraction of the gallbladder that squirts the concentrated liquid bile into the small intestine where it helps with the emulsification of fats in the meal.

Bile is a bitter, yellow fluid. It can consist of cholesterol, lecithin, calcium, bile salts, acids and waste materials among other things. Gallstones are formed when bile salts and cholesterol levels become imbalanced. Bile is continually being made and secreted by the liver into bile ducts in varying amounts.

Bile has two major functions in the body. First, it breaks down the fats from the diet so that the body can utilize them. Without adequate bile we are not able to metabolize fats, which can result in a deficiency of the fat-soluble vitamins A, D, E and K. Insufficient bile also inhibits the metabolizing of essential fatty acids and the body's utilization of calcium. Physical signs of inefficient bile are dry skin and peeling on the soles of the feet.

You can tell you have trouble digesting fats if you have excessive burping that starts shortly after eating a meal that has fat in it. You might feel nauseous or experience gas and bloating. Some people also may get diarrhea if they ingest a fatty meal.

Bile's second function is to serve as a powerful antioxidant that helps to remove toxins from the liver. The pathway of digestive departure is from the liver through the bile ducts and into the gallbladder or directly into the small intestine where it joins waste matter and leaves through the colon with the feces. Many of our used up or metabolized hormones get excreted through the bile such as estrogen and steroid hormones such as cortisol. The digestive system relies on good bile flow to assist with ridding the body of used up hormones.

THE LIVER

The liver, for lack of a better description, is the body's master filter performing many functions that are vital to life. The liver plays a crucial role in digestion (breaking down of nutrients) and assimilation (putting nutrients to use). The liver is the storage site for many essential vitamins and minerals such as iron, copper, B12 and vitamins A, D, E and K. The liver even produces red blood cells and Kupffer cells to help devour harmful microorganisms in the blood to fight infection.

The liver is one of the most important organs in the body with regard to detoxification, especially from the gut. The liver utilizes most of the body's nutrition (vitamins, minerals and compounds found in food) to perform its detoxification function. The liver detoxifies harmful substances through a complex series of chemical reactions using enzymes, co-factors (vitamins) and nutrients to neutralize the toxin and excrete it through urine or bile.

Many of the toxic chemicals that enter the body are fat-soluble, which means they dissolve only in fatty or oily solutions and not in water. This makes the toxin difficult for the body to excrete. Fat-soluble chemicals have a high affinity for fat tissues and cell membranes, which are composed of fatty acids and proteins.

So what does your body do with toxins it cannot detoxify? Unfortunately, it keeps them. The body stores the toxins right in the fat cells on your butt, hips and belly. There is a lot more "junk in your trunk" than you may have thought. Fatty tissues of the body are the preferred waste dumps for toxins. These fatty tissues may hold on to these toxins for years, only to be released during times of exercise, stress or fasting. During the release of these toxins, symptoms such as headaches, poor memory, stomach pain, nausea, fatigue, dizziness and palpitations may occur.

Much of the blood being filtered by the liver is from the portal vein carrying blood from the intestines. The liver acts as a virtual bug catcher removing a broad spectrum of microorganisms such as bacteria, fungi, viruses and parasites from the blood. You certainly do not want these building up in the blood and invading deeper parts of the body.

The body's normal metabolic processes produce a wide range of chemicals and hormones all of which the liver is able to neutralize. However, the level and type of internally produced toxins increases greatly when metabolic processes go awry, typically as a result of nutritional deficiencies (e.g., a bad diet).

Many of the toxic chemicals the liver must detoxify come from the environment: the content of the bowels, food, water and air and soil pollution. Herbicides and pesticides are just one example of chemicals that are now found in virtually all fat tissues of the human body. Even if you eat unprocessed, organic foods, your liver will have to detoxify because all foods contain naturally occurring toxic constituents.

The liver plays several roles in detoxification: 1) it filters the blood to remove toxins; 2) it synthesizes and secretes bile full of cholesterol and other fat-soluble toxins; and 3) it enzymatically breaks down unwanted chemicals. The enzymatic process performed by the liver occurs in two phases: phase I and phase II. Phase I either directly neutralizes a toxin, or modifies the toxic chemical to form activated intermediates that are then neutralized by one or more of the several phase II enzyme systems.

If you are still contemplating the importance of the liver in the detoxification process, consider this: 75 percent of nutrition contributes to the liver detoxification process; up to 90 percent of all cancers are thought to be due to the effects of environmental toxins, such as those in cigarette smoke, food, water and air combined with nutrition deficiencies necessary for proper functioning of the detoxification and immune systems. The level of exposure to environmental carcinogens varies widely, as does the efficiency of the detoxification enzymes, particularly phase II.

When optimum nutrition is provided, the liver operates efficiently. If nutrition is compromised through poor dietary and lifestyle habits, detoxification processes are compromised and other organs suffer as the body retains these toxins.

ADDITIONAL FUNCTIONS OF THE LIVER

Filtering the Blood

One of the liver's primary functions is filtering the blood. When working properly, the liver clears 99 percent of the bacteria and other toxins during the first pass. However, when the liver is damaged, the passage of toxins increases.

Bile Secretion

The liver's second detoxification process involves the creation and secretion of bile. Each day the liver manufactures approximately one quart of bile that serves as a carrier for the many toxic substances being dumped into the intestines. In the intestines, the bile and its toxic load are absorbed by fiber and then excreted. However, a diet low in fiber results in inadequate binding and re-absorption of the toxins.

PHASE I DETOXIFICATION

The liver's third role in detoxification involves a two-step enzymatic process for the neutralization of unwanted chemical compounds. This pathway converts toxic chemicals into less harmful chemicals. Free radicals are produced during the process; however, excessive production of free radicals can damage the liver cells. Antioxidants reduce the damage caused by free radicals. If antioxidants are lacking and toxin exposure is high, toxic chemicals get a shuttle bus with a one-way ticket to your fat cells.

People with underactive phase I detoxification will often experience multiple chemical sensitivities: caffeine intolerance, as well as intolerances to perfumes and other environmental chemicals. Being overly sensitive to chemicals or extremely sensitive to the caffeine in coffee is a marker of probable impairment phase I detoxification.

Toxin sensitivities are different from person to person. The body uses enzymes to detoxify certain types of chemicals, and the enzymes often work together to detoxify the body. The group of enzymes in phase I detoxification are collectively called cytochrome P450. Cytochrome P450 are a group of enzymes that combine oxygen with iron to release hydrogen, often as part of the body's strategy to dispose of potentially harmful substances by making them more water-soluble. Just as a metal roof rusts from exposure to the environment, our toxins in the body can become "rusted" from the detoxification process.

The activity of the various cytochrome P450 enzymes varies significantly from one individual to another based on the person's genetics, the level of exposure to toxins and the person's nutritional status. Since the activity of cytochrome P450 varies so greatly, the individual's ability to detoxify will either increase or decrease his or her risk for various diseases.

When the cytochrome P450 enzymes metabolize a toxin, the toxin chemically transforms either into a less toxic form making it water-soluble and therefore able to excrete through the kidney, or in some cases, the enzymes convert the toxin to a more chemically reactive form, allowing the toxin to become more easily metabolized by the phase II enzymes.

A significant side effect of phase I detoxification is the production of free radicals as the toxins are starting to be broken down. For each molecule of toxin metabolized by phase I, one molecule of free radical is generated from the oxidization, or "rusting," process. Without adequate free radical defenses, every time the liver neutralizes a toxin exposure a free radical may go on to damage the body.

The toxins transformed into intermediate substances by phase I are often substantially more reactive than the original toxins. Therefore, the rate at which phase I produces intermediates must be balanced by the rate at which phase II finishes their processing—meaning the cycle of phase I detoxification must be balanced with the cycle of phase II. Think of it this way: depositing money in your bank account (phase 2) must be moving at the same rate of speed or faster than the speed in which you write checks (phase 1), or you will have a serious build up of insufficient fund letters (toxins) in your mailbox (fat cells).

If you have a very active phase I detoxification system coupled with slow or inactive phase II enzymes, you will most likely suffer unusually high toxic reactions to environmental poisons. There are several ways to test liver function. My preferred method of testing is the organic acid test, which pinpoints exactly how efficiently the liver is carrying out the detoxification process.

An imbalance between phase I and phase II can also occur when a person is exposed to large amounts of toxins or exposed to toxins for a long period of time. In these situations, the critical nutrients needed for phase II detoxification are depleted allowing the highly toxic, activated intermediates to build up.

An efficient liver detoxification system is vital to health. In order to support this process, it is essential that many key nutrients are included in the diet. The following vitamins play a significant role in phase I detoxification:

- B Vitamins: The B vitamins play a major role in detoxification acting as cofactors for many enzyme systems including those of liver detoxification. Obviously, ensuring a plentiful supply of the B complex group of vitamins is of prime importance for optimum detoxification.
- Vitamin C: Vitamin C prevents free radical formation.
- Vitamin E and selenium: Vitamin E and selenium are cofactors for glutathione activity as well as being powerful antioxidants.
- Other nutrients that play vital roles in the phase II pathway include the following amino acids from proteins: glycine, cysteine, glutamine, methionine, taurine, glutamic acid and aspartic acid.

Recent research shows that the cytochrome P450 enzyme systems are also found in other parts of the body, especially the brain cells. Inadequate antioxidants and nutrients in the brain result in an increased rate of neuron damage as seen in Alzheimer's and Parkinson's disease patients. As with all enzymes, the cytochrome P450 enzymes require several nutrients to function (copper, magnesium, zinc and vitamin C). A considerable amount of research has found that various substances activate cytochrome P450 while others inhibit it.

Among foods, the brassica family such as cabbage, broccoli, and brussels sprouts, contains chemical constituents that stimulate both phase I and phase II detoxification enzymes. So yes, your mom was right. You do need to eat your broccoli!

Oranges, lemons, limes and tangerines as well as the seeds of caraway and dill contain limonene, a phytochemical that has been found to prevent and even treat cancer in animal models. Limonene's protective effects are probably due to the fact that it is a strong inducer of both phase I and phase II detoxification enzymes that neutralize carcinogens. The following substances activate phase I detoxification:

- Drugs: alcohol, nicotine, Phenobarbital, sulfonamides and steroids
- Foods: cabbage, broccoli and brussels sprouts; charcoal-broiled meats; high-protein diet; oranges and tangerines (but not grapefruits)
- Nutrients: niacin, vitamin B1 and vitamin C

- Environmental toxins: carbon tetrachloride, exhaust fumes, paint fumes, dioxin and pesticides

INHIBITORS OF PHASE I DETOXIFICATION

Many substances inhibit or slow the actions of the phase I cytochrome P450 enzymes, which slows the body's ability to rid itself of toxins. The longer the toxins reside in the body, the more toxic they become.

- Drugs: benzodiazepines, antihistamines, cimetidine and other antacids, ketoconazole and sulfaphenazole
- Foods: naringenin from grapefruit juice; *curcumin from turmeric; capsaicin form chili pepper; eugenol from clove oil; and quercetin from onions
- Botanicals: curcuma longa (curcumin); capsicum frutescens (capsaicin); eugenia caryophyllus (eugenol); calendula officianalis

* Aging Toxins from inappropriate bacteria in the intestines

*Curcumin, the compound that gives turmeric its yellow color, inhibits phase I while stimulating phase II.

*The activity of phase I detoxification enzymes decreases as we age. Aging also decreases blood flow through the liver, further aggravating the problem. The lack of adequate physical activity necessary for good circulation paired with the poor nutrition combine to create a significant impairment of detoxification capacity.

PHASE II DETOXIFICATION

Phase II detoxification is referred to as the conjugation, or the "coupling," pathway, whereby the liver cells add another substance (i.e., cysteine, glycine or a sulphur molecule) to a toxic chemical or drug rendering it less harmful. Through conjugation, the liver is able to turn drugs, hormones and various toxins into substances capable of excretion.

The liver cells require sulphur-containing amino acids such as taurine and cysteine and glycine, glutamine, choline and inositol for efficient phase II detoxification. Phase II detoxification is comprised of seven pathways.

THE SEVEN PATHWAYS OF PHASE II DETOXIFICATION

Pathway 1: Glutathione Conjugation

Conjugation, joining a toxin with a substance, with glutathione is a primary phase II detoxification pathway. Glutathione conjugation produces water-soluble metabolites that are excreted from the kidneys. Glutathione is the master antioxidant and is produced by the body in every cell. Glutathione is one of the most important anti-carcinogens and antioxidants in the body's cells. A glutathione deficiency can cause serious liver dysfunction and damage.

The elimination of fat-soluble compounds, especially heavy metals such as mercury and lead, is dependent upon adequate levels of glutathione, which in turn is dependent upon adequate levels of methionine and cysteine from the diet or supplementation.

Pathway 2: Amino Acid Conjugation

Several amino acids from the diet including glycine, taurine, glutamine, arginine and ornithine are used to combine with dietary proteins and neutralize toxins. Of these, glycine is the most commonly utilized in phase II amino acid detoxification.

Even in normal adults, a wide variation exists in the activity of the glycine conjugation pathway. This is due not only to genetic variation, but also to the availability of glycine in the liver. Glycine, and the other amino acids used for conjugation, becomes deficient on a low-protein diet as well as from chronic exposure to toxins.

Pathway 3: Methylation

Methylation involves detoxifying steroid hormones such as estrogen. Most of the methyl groups used for detoxification come from sadenosylmethionine (SAM). The process of creating SAM requires the amino acid methionine, the nutrients choline, the active form of B12 (methylcobalamin), which by the way requires sufficient stomach acid for absorption, and the active folic acid (5-methyltetrahydrofolate). Vitally important to women, SAM is able to inactivate estrogens (through methylation), supporting the use of methionine in conditions of estrogen excess such as premenstrual syndrome.

Pathway 4: Sulfation

Sulfation is the main pathway for detoxifying cortisol as well as food additives, environmental toxins and prescription drugs. Sulfation is also the primary route for the elimination of used neurotransmitters such as serotonin and norepinephrine.

Pathway 5: Acetylation

Acetylation is the process of binding toxins with acetyl-CoA. It is the primary method by which the body eliminates sulfa drugs such as Septra and Bactrim. This system appears to be especially sensitive to genetic variation with those having a poor acetylation system being far more susceptible to adverse reactions to sulfa drugs and other antibiotics.

Pathway 6: Glucuronidation

Glucuronidation is the combining of glucuronic acid with toxins. Many of the commonly prescribed drugs are detoxified through this pathway. It also helps to detoxify aspirin, menthol, food additives such as benzoates and some hormones. Calcium d-glucarate, a natural ingredient found in certain foods such as apples and brussels sprouts may increase elimination of toxins through glucuronidation.

Pathway 7: Sulfoxidation

Sulfoxidation is the process by which the sulfur-containing molecules in drugs and foods are metabolized. It is also the process by which the body eliminates the sulfite food additives used to preserve many foods and drugs. Normally, the enzyme sulfiteoxidase metabolizes sulfites to the safer sulfates, which are then excreted in the urine. People who have a poorly functioning sulfoxidation system are more sensitive to sulfur-containing drugs and foods containing sulfur or sulfite additives. So, if you get a headache from red wine, you may have a slow sulfoxidation process.

The following nutrients are required for the proper functioning of phase II detoxification enzymes:

- Glutathione conjugation: glutathione precursors (cysteine, glycine, glutamic acid and co-factors), omega-3 and -6 essential fatty acids
- Amino acid conjugation: glycine
- Methylation: methionine and co-factors (magnesium, folic acid, B-12, SAM)
- Sulfation: molybdenum, cysteine and precursor (methionine), co-factors (B-12, folic acid, magnesium and B-6/ pyridoxal-5'-phosphate) and MSM
- Acetylation: acetyl-CoA, molybdenum, iron, B-3 (niacinamide), B-2 (riboflavin)
- Glucuronidation: glucuronic acid and magnesium

- Glycination: arginase enzyme, glycine, gly co-factors (folic acid, manganese, B-2, the active form of B-6 called P-5-P)

The following are inducers of phase II detoxification:

- Glutathione conjugation: brassica family foods (cabbage, broccoli, brussels sprouts) and limonene-containing foods (citrus peel, dill weed oil and caraway oil)
- Sulfation: taurine and the amino acids cysteine and methionine
- Acetylation: none
- Amino acid conjugation: glycine
- Methylation: lipotropic nutrients (choline, methionine, betaine, folic acid and vitamin B12)
- Glucuronidation: fish oils and limonene-containing foods

The following are inhibitors of phase II inducers of phase II detoxification enzymes:

- Glutathione conjugation: selenium deficiency, vitamin B2 deficiency, glutathione deficiency and zinc deficiency
- Amino acid conjugation: low protein diet
- Methylation: folic acid or vitamin B12 deficiency
- Sulfation: non-steroidal, anti-inflammatory drugs (e.g., aspirin), tartrazine (yellow food dye) and molybdenum deficiency
- Acetylation: vitamin B2, B5 or C deficiency
- Glucuronidation: aspirin and probenecid

Bile Excretion

One of the primary routes for the elimination of modified toxins from the liver is through the bile. Impairment of bile flow within the liver can be caused by a variety of agents and conditions. These conditions are often associated with alterations of liver function in laboratory tests (serum bilirubin, alkaline phosphatase, SGOT, LDH, GGTP, etc.) signifying cellular damage. However, relying on these tests alone to evaluate liver function is not adequate, since, in the initial or subclinical stages of many problems with liver function, laboratory values remain normal. Non-standard laboratory tests such as organic acid testing from urine can detect functional errors in detoxification even when blood levels of liver enzymes such as SGOT and AST (serum glutamic-oxaloacetic transaminase and aspartate aminotransferase, respectively) are normal. Among the symptoms people with enzymatic damage complain of are fatigue, general malaise, digestive disturbances, allergies and chemical sensitivities, premenstrual syndrome and constipation.

Nutritional Factors of Liver Detoxification Support

Antioxidant vitamins such vitamin C, beta-carotene and vitamin E are obviously quite important in protecting the liver from damage as well as helping in the detoxification mechanisms, but even simple nutrients such as B-vitamins, calcium and trace minerals are critical in the elimination of heavy metals and other toxic compounds from the body. The lipotropic agents such as choline, betaine, methionine, vitamin B6, folic acid and vitamin B12 are useful as they promote the flow of fat and bile to and from the liver.

In healthy individuals, a daily dosage of 800 mg of vitamin C with N-acetylcysteine (NAC), glycine and methionine can improve cellular glutathione levels.

Botanical Medicines

There is a long list of plants that exert beneficial effects on liver function. However, the most impressive research has been done on silymarin, the flavonoids extracted from silybum marianum (milk thistle). These compounds exert a substantial effect on protecting the liver from damage as well as enhancing the detoxification processes. Silymarin prevents damage to the liver through several mechanisms: acting as an antioxidant; increasing the synthesis of glutathione; and increasing the rate of liver tissue regeneration.

Silymarin is many times more potent in antioxidant activity than vitamin E and vitamin C. The protective effect of silymarin against liver damage has been demonstrated in numerous experimental studies. One of the key mechanisms by which silymarin enhances detoxification is by preventing the depletion of glutathione.

Another significantly studied compound in foods that has shown promise in both detoxification and cancer prevention is sulforaphane. Sulforaphane is a compound that was identified in broccoli sprouts by researchers investigating the anti-cancer compounds present in broccoli. They discovered that broccoli sprouts contain anywhere from 30 to 50 times the concentration of protective chemicals that are found in mature broccoli plants. Sulforaphane is an antioxidant and potent stimulator of natural detoxifying enzymes in the body. Foods that contain sulforaphane are broccoli and other cruciferous vegetables such as cauliflower, cabbage and kale.

Feeding sulforaphane-rich broccoli sprout extracts to laboratory rats exposed to cancer-causing chemicals dramatically reduced the frequency, size and number of the rats' tumors. Human studies with sulforaphane and other cruciferous-vegetable components have shown that these compounds stimulate the body's production of detoxification enzymes and exert antioxidant effects.

Preliminary studies suggest that in order to cut the risk of cancer in half, the average person would need to eat about two pounds of broccoli or similar vegetables per week. Since the concentration of sulforaphane is much higher in broccoli sprouts than in mature broccoli, the same reduction in risk theoretically might be had with a weekly intake of just over an ounce of sprouts. Eat that broccoli!

Foods

Foods such as vegetables, fruit and whole unprocessed grains are vital to provide the right nutritional content such as vitamin C, beta-carotene and vitamin E. It is also very important to the liver detoxification process that you get adequate protein that provides the full array of amino acids such as glycine, methionine, B-12, cysteine and methionine.

Whew! The liver is one busy organ!

FUNCTIONS OF THE LYMPHATIC SYSTEM

The lymphatic system plays a major role in our immune system's defense against infection and cancer. This system consists of vessels connected to several lymph nodes and draws fluid into and out of the bloodstream. The lymph nodes act as filters that contain many lymphocytes or white blood cells that destroy bacteria and viruses. While helping to fight infection, the lymph nodes may become swollen and tender much like when you get a sore throat.

Another function of the lymphatic system is the absorption of fats and proteins from our daily diet through the intestinal walls, which gives the lymph fluid its milky color. The lymph fluid is circulated by the movement of our muscles through a system of one-way valves.

Unlike the circulatory system, the lymphatic system has no pump, so the more of a couch potato you are the more likely it that your lymphatic system is congested. Lack of exercise reduces circulation, and thus the transfer of oxygen to the cells. This leads to high blood pressure and fluid retention.

The lack of adenosine tri-phosphate (ATP) causes the glucose in the cells to ferment creating an anaerobic (without oxygen) condition. An anaerobic condition upsets the metabolic processes of the cell. These cells, lacking sufficient oxygen, soon become weak and unhealthy. If prolonged, the entire immune system may start breaking down.

ATP is created from the chemical reactions between glucose and oxygen, which is required for all the energy requiring reactions of cellular metabolism. Glucose or sugars are the fuel for the cells and the ATP is the energy. Foods that contain high amounts of oxygen are complex carbohydrates such as fresh raw fruits and vegetables, whole grains, seeds and nuts.

The lymphatic system is much like a janitorial service. It helps get oxygen and nutrients to the cells by removing dead cells, poisons, toxins and excess water from the tissue spaces around the cells. All of our body tissue cells are bathed in this fluid, or extra-cellular water, derived from our bloodstream. In fact, our blood is about 92 percent water. Eventually the lymph fluid makes its way into the thoracic duct just under the clavicle bones and drains into the subclavian veins and into the heart.

A slow moving lymphatic system, intestinal problems and poor diet may cause excess lymph fluid water around tissue cells increasing the potential for disease, infection, cancer and oxygen deficiency. Intestinal tract cleansing helps the absorption of nutrients and fats needed for correct lymphatic system functioning. Eating fresh fruits and vegetables helps raise oxygen, energy and nutrient levels.

Remedies for a Slow-Mo Lymphatic System

The nutrients we feed our body via fresh foods are potential energy. These nutrients are changed into chemical energy with oxygen through the oxidative process converting potential energy into actual life in the cells. Eating junk food forces us to use up more of its oxygen reserves than usual in order to metabolize the preservatives and what few nutrients may actually be in the food.

Foods such as fats and proteins are not only low in oxygen content, but also require extra oxygen from our bodies to convert them into energy, which further depletes our oxygen reserves. Other oxygen-robbing foods include processed sugar, white flour, alcohol, coffee and soda drinks.

Some drugs have calcium and potassium blockers that cause other problems. Some of the prescription drugs used for high blood pressure will cause excess fluid retention around the cell tissue as well as other problems. Garlic works well for high blood pressure. Herbs that work as diuretics are astragalus, chaparral, corn silk, dandelion, gotu kola, horsetail, juniper berries, nettle, parsley and uva ursi, as well as vitamin B6 and the amino acid arginine, which help to reduce water retention and improve lymphatic function.

Also, as you may have guessed, regular physical movement that is aerobic in nature is beneficial as well because it increases oxygen utilization. Exercise also increases muscular contraction, which moves the lymph system, and even makes you sweat thereby removing even more toxins in the process.

LUNGS

The lungs are responsible for delivering oxygen to the blood. For that reason, they are exposed to toxic environmental pollutants and play a role in the health of your body. The following factors contribute to poor lung functioning: a poor diet, living in a polluted area, shallow breathing and smoking. When the lungs are not functionally optimally, the body experiences a reduction in the amount of circulating oxygen, and consequently a reduction in the amount of carbon dioxide that is exhaled from the body. By supporting the lungs with good nutrition and by learning breathing techniques, we can effectively cleanse the lungs allowing for better functioning.

DEEP BREATHING EXERCISE

Learning deep breathing is an important aspect of lung detoxification. One example of this is belly breathing: inhale through the nose trying to pull the air down to your belly. You cannot physically breathe into the belly, but you can cause the lungs to expand down instead of out by pulling the diaphragm down. Once you completely fill the lungs from the bottom up, exhale slowly through the nose and mouth. Allow the exhaling to take longer than the inhaling.

Detoxifying the lungs starts with breathing clean air and breathing deeply. Include as many cruciferous, green vegetables as possible in the diet, as this can actually help to detoxify, support and heal the lungs.

SKIN

Our skin is a very busy organ, excreting waste and even generating nutrients such as vitamin D. The skin is the largest organ of the body. The skin performs the following functions: temperature regulation, regulation of fluid absorption, and the secretion of an acidic substance that inhibits bacteria and excretion of waste materials via the sweat glands. In fact, some toxic heavy metals are also released from the body when we sweat. The sweat glands of the skin can perform as much detoxification as one kidney. Therefore, it is important for the skin to be maintained so that it can perform detoxification at maximum levels. The detoxification function of the skin is especially important if someone has damaged kidneys.

The skin is permeable, meaning it will absorb what it is expose it to. Therefore, the use of synthetic and chemical laden skin care, cleaning, laundry and dry cleaning are not good. These chemicals can be absorbed into the circulatory system through the skin providing more toxins to the body. Most people do not feel the ill effects of these chemical additives instantly, because most of the time, the liver is able to metabolize and detoxify them. However, people who are sensitive, or especially toxic, can quickly become sick from these chemicals.

Because the skin absorbs the chemicals it comes in contact with, it is important to provide the right environment for your skin: clean your skin using natural soaps; moisturize using all natural, no preservative moisturizers; and use all natural, no preservative foundation make-up and powder. Wear clothes with natural fibers such as organic cotton and flax.

Proper nutrition is also important for the skin. Our skin is mainly fat so it is wise to eat high quality fats from a natural origin. Olive oil, flax, fish oils and real butter are great sources of natural fats and oils that can help maintain healthy skin from the inside out. Proper hydration will also alleviate dry skin.

Benefits of sweating as a natural skin detoxifier:

- Sweating via heat treatments such as saunas or sweaty exercises allow a rise in body temperature that causes peripheral circulatory dilation and reduction in blood pressure while excreting waste through sweating.
- Sweating via a source of heat causes the loss of water, salt, urea, uric acid, sulfates, creatinine, phosphates and lactic acid.
- Sweating increases the metabolism and stimulates the immune system.

- Sweating increases oxygen availability to the body, decreasing lymphatic congestion and removes selected heavy metals.
- Sweating restores the natural pH of the skin and hair.
- Sweating decrease toxins inside the body.
- Sweating has sedating and relaxing effects on the body.

Beyond being the veil we show to the outside world, our skin is a very busy organ and deserves our attention and care. Take time while on The Cleanse Program to get some sweaty exercise, hydrate and care for your skin with natural products, and you will see the difference.

9
Conscious Cleansing

> *The greatest discovery of my generation is that a human being can alter his life by altering his attitudes of mind. - William James*

KELLYE HOWELL, TESTIMONIAL

I have been a health advocate for years. I am an avid runner, skier and vegetarian with a serious interest in staying healthy. My friend wanted a partner to do The Cleanse Program with so I decided I would do it with her. I figured, since my diet was already really good, I would pick up a few tidbits of new information and would provide the support for my dear friend.

Even though I had a pretty balanced diet before The Cleanse Program, I did experience energy fluctuation throughout the day and consumed too much sugar and sweets in my diet. Getting off of the sugar had a profound effect on my energy.

I also noticed that my digestion was much better and the bloating and mild discomfort I had become accustomed to was gone. Before the cleanse, I did not know my digestion issues were abnormal or unusual. Sometimes you have to get better before you know you have an issue! When I went through the reintroduction of foods, I found that grains containing gluten was the culprit in the bloating and slow digestion.

As a result of The Cleanse Program, I have removed gluten from my diet, and my digestion works in tiptop shape. I also learned that dairy and corn are foods I need to eat sparingly. I enjoy using many of the "cleanse" recipes and have also incorporated the cleaning product recipes.

NURTURE OR NOURISH?

Toxic Emotions & Food

People engage in a detox program for many reasons, one of which is to jumpstart a weight loss program. Before starting a new dietary regime, it is important to take a close look at how and why we eat. It should come as no surprise that most of us eat for many reasons other than nourishment. We eat because it is social. We eat to combat stress. We eat for a quick pick-me-up—think about those late afternoon chocolate cravings. We eat for innumerable reasons outside of nourishment.

Many people may honestly believe that they only eat when they are hungry and never at any other time or for any other reason. So when you are watching that football game, is it really necessary to have the nachos and the corn dogs? What about popcorn at the movie, or a pint of ice cream when your dating life is not going as smoothly as you would like? Is the peppermint latte really because you are hungry? You can probably think of many occasions in which you have eaten for a reason other than nourishment. You may even be able to think of something you ate today that falls into the "nurture not nourish" category.

Many times we are completely aware of what we are doing, and we consciously pick and choose what we are eating. Other times, we are not quite so aware, and this is when we unintentionally use food medicinally.

In order to get the most from your cleanse experience, you really need to explore the emotional terrain of your eating habits. For instance, perhaps you are mad today, so you decide that you deserve a chocolate sundae. Or, maybe you are dining on an expense account and someone else is paying for your food—you may choose to have a steak, a glass of wine, etc. When these types of thoughts occur, you are using food inappropriately. Sadness, anger, loneliness, boredom—these are all toxic emotions that can lead to emotional eating.

Boredom is an especially toxic emotion for people who spend their workday in a cubicle or chained to a desk. If you have ever worked in a cubicle you have probably found yourself wandering at one time or another from cube to cube looking for whatever someone else may have to snack on. In these moments, chances are you are bored, unchallenged and perhaps even a little angry, but you probably are not actually hungry.

Becoming aware of the emotions you are experiencing when you eat is very important. Only when we are aware if our emotions can we catch ourselves in the action of emotional eating.

Taking control of emotional eating can be challenging because it is difficult to identify the action while in the moment. Many people are not taught at an early age to express their emotions properly, if at all. Sometimes we have been taught to only identify and express "positive" feelings and to bury the "negative" feelings such as pain, sadness, depression, loss, anxiety and other very real and often helpful emotions. You may have been taught that outward displays of feelings are taboo, or perhaps the opposite is true. You may have been raised in an environment where there was so much display of emotions that you do not want any part of it.

A healthy relationship with food is one in which food has no emotion attached to it. So, how do you get to a place where your relationship with food is neither good nor bad, and where your emotional reaction to food is neutral? The first step is to identify your feelings as you experience them, and then rank them in order of intensity. For example, you may feel sad or bored, which can be the same thing, but can also be slightly different. Which emotion is more intense? This is an important exercise in taking control of your emotional eating. Next, make a list of the feelings you really hate to experience. Many women are taught that it is wrong to have feelings of anger or rage. In actuality, it is not the feeling that is wrong, but the inappropriate expressions of such feelings. Feelings are not appropriate or inappropriate; they are simply emotions. It is how we choose to express or repress our emotions that can be inappropriate.

Food is often a drug of choice. Some people drink. Some people do drugs, smoke or gamble. Some people medicate their emotions with food. During The Cleanse Program, you may tap into your demons, so to speak, as you start cleaning up your diet and lifestyle, which makes this is a good time to address the emotional aspect of eating as well. If you think you may struggle with using food as a drug, I recommend following the exercise.

Are you aware that in any given moment you may have multiple feelings at once? Can you name those feelings? Can you rank them in order of intensity or in order of comfort (or discomfort)? If so, rank your feelings from most comfortable to the least comfortable. Make a list of the top five feelings you experience the most intensely.

Most people can name only one feeling at a time, or we have no idea what we are feeling unless it is extreme. How can we be so unaware of what we are feeling if emotions are such a regular part of our daily existence? There are two reasons: 1) We have not been taught to identify what we are feeling, and 2) we are afraid of our feelings. We learn these traits from both our families and from our culture.

Good feelings like joy, happiness, strong, beautiful and healthy can also lead to a more positive outlook and better food choices. Often when we feel good about ourselves and our lives we have a pep in our step and pick vibrant, vital and alive foods.

On the other hand, most of us have feelings that we consider "bad" feelings. These are the ones that are so painful or difficult to face that we do whatever we can to eliminate or kill them. For many of us, food is the drug that does the killing. When we start to feel the "bad" feeling, we eat, and then the feeling subsides. When the feeling comes back, we eat again.

A significant step to managing feelings, and that often leads to managing eating, is learning to identify the emotions you eat to kill. Below are the ten most toxic emotions that most people have difficulty handling. You will probably find that simply reading this list will bring up undesirable emotions within you. All of us have some of these feelings some of the time, but we ignore or suppress them.

The Nasty Feelings We Eat to Kill

- Guilt
- Hurt
- Loneliness
- Self-loathing
- Anger
- Anxiety
- Deprivation
- Disappointment
- Emptiness
- Sadness

If you don't see your "favorite" nasty feeling on the list, write it in the margin. The only way to overcome emotional eating is to first know what you are feeling. The truth is that many feelings come in powerful toxic duos or trios that are extremely difficult to identify and manage. For instance, self-loathing, guilt and hurt are a common toxic trio. Another common combination is deprivation and emptiness. Disappointment, hurt and sadness are also common partners.

No wonder we have so much trouble controlling emotional eating! No wonder so many diets do not work. If you have little to no ability to identify and manage these powerful feelings, you are often at their mercy. You can manage these feelings by controlling your eating habits.

The first step to identifying the emotion is to simply "sit" with the feeling. Maybe choose one feeling from the list above. Close your eyes and remember a time you felt that feeling. Try to recall as much detail as possible: the scenario, the people involved, and what was said or done. Second, just feel the emotions as they arise. Sit with them. Next, choose a feeling that you enjoy feeling (obviously not on the list). Remember a time you felt that feeling, and try to recall as much about what happened when you experienced that emotion. Enjoy yourself, and when you are ready, open your eyes.

What did you notice? In this short exercise, you were able to change how you felt by just thinking differently. In the first step, you thought of a bad situation, felt the feelings associated with that and literally re-experienced the situation. In the second situation, you felt completely different and better. Obviously, we have the power to change our emotions by changing how we think and what we think about.

Now that we know this little tidbit of information, we can use it to our advantage to get a handle on emotional eating. During The Cleanse Program, try to identify your triggers to eat when you are not physically hungry (usually an empty feeling in the pit of the stomach). Go through the exercise above to see if you can reset your emotions.

USE THE CLEANSE PROGRAM TO DEVELOP A NEW RELATIONSHIP WITH FOOD

Going on The Cleanse Program often brings up many feelings and may even uncover hidden feelings about food, particularly overeating and emotional eating. While on The Cleanse Program, try this experiment to begin understanding your relationship with fullness. To start this process, start eating before you feel famished and only eat until you are satisfied or less than full.

Fullness Scale

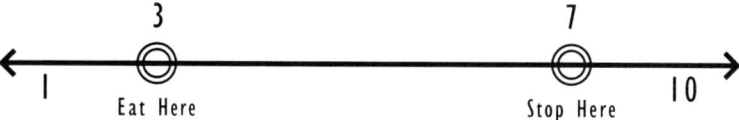

Eat till you are at about a three on a scale of one to ten, with one being starving and ten being stuffed to the max. How do you know when you are at a three? Most people feel true hunger in the stomach region as a feeling of empty or a slight ache. If you feel famished, light-headed or cannot think straight without eating, you have gone too far.

Eat until you are about a seven on the same scale. Eat until you are partially full but not uncomfortable. How do you know you are at a seven? If you are eating slowly and mindfully, you will notice small physical sensations that culminate in a sense of fullness when you are finished eating.

During the next few weeks, know that you can eat at any time if you are physically hungry and stay within the comfort range—you can always have more later (today, tomorrow, next week, next year, etc.). We often mistakenly believe that the food is "so good" that we will never be able to eat it again. Ninety-ninety percent of the time, that is not even possible. We could buy it again, make it again, and eat at the restaurant again at any time.

Our moms were wrong! We are not saving any starving children by cleaning our plates; we are just adding fat to our bellies when we eat too much. Over the next week, keep a food log recording your eating experiences: How hungry were you when you ate? How full were you when you finished? How did you feel emotionally prior to eating as well as after?

EXAMPLE

Guideline: I will eat when I am at a three on the scale and finish eating at a seven.

I thought about eating when I was at a three but got distracted and waited too long to eat. I found it hard to manage my hunger. I made choices I did not originally want to make. I learned that waiting until I was famished was leading to overeating at my next meal.

Guideline Log 1

_____
_____
_____
_____
_____

Guideline Log 2

Guideline Log 3

Guideline Log 4

Guideline Log 5

_____
_____
_____
_____
_____
_____
_____

Guideline Log 6

_____
_____
_____
_____
_____
_____
_____

Guideline Log 7

_____
_____
_____
_____
_____
_____
_____

Review your log and determine the three overriding messages that may not actually be helping you to achieve your detox goals. By looking back, you will often find common reasons for why you may overeat, or why you may choose unhealthy foods to eat such as ignoring your body's signals or eating when you really are craving love or affection. You can work on these negative feeling messages by reframing or rewording these messages to be more empowering.

EXAMPLE

Message: By noticing that your eating may be motivated by a need for feeling love, your message of "food is love" may change to "food is fuel and nourishment." This demonstrates a healthy reframing of food. Food does not provide love. A healthy relationship with oneself and others provides love. Now, you do it. Reframe your messages to be a more empowering message!

Message 1

_____
_____
_____
_____
_____

Message 2

_____
_____
_____
_____
_____

Message 3

_____
_____
_____
_____
_____

CLEANSE STRESS BY PRACTICING MINDFUL EATING

The Cleanse Program is more than just a physical body cleanse. We are going to cleanse the mind as well. By becoming more in tune with how your body signals, you will find that you are able to actually reduce your stress. One way to really kick this process up a notch is to practice mindful eating. Mindful eating refers to the innate internal cues we experience that inform our bodies that we are hungry (and if so, how hungry) or satiated in order to guide our eating. As infants, we naturally followed these cues; however, as schedules and rules were implemented, we learned to distrust our cues. As we grew from children to teens and then on to adulthood, our attitudes about food became molded by societal and familial norms and expectations. As humans, our relationship with food shifts very early in life from simply being a source of nutrition to becoming a source of comfort and sometimes a source of pain. Periodic bouts of dieting—for some people, even living on a diet—and living in constant fear that what we eat will make us fat skews our understanding and relationship with food. Mindful eating is positive. Mindful eating is an essential part of living well and leading a healthy lifestyle.

What is Mindful Eating?

Mindful eating is eating in a supportive manner, using our bodies' cues or messages such as fullness and physical hunger to guide us in what, when and how much we should eat for satisfaction and health. Mindful eating includes all types of foods that make us feel well, but that can vary from time to time as well as from person to person.

Strategies for Eating Mindfully

Eat when you are hungry. Watch for your body's hunger cues as your signal that it is time to eat. Remember what you learned during the fullness exercises about hunger and fullness. Most people feel true physical hunger in their stomachs. Watch for where you feel hungry. If it is not in the stomach, ask yourself if you are hungry for something non-food related.

Don't let yourself get too hungry. The goal is to eat when you are about 30 percent hungry and to stop eating when you are 70 percent full—satisfied and comfortably full, not stuffed.

Eat balanced meals. A balanced meal should include protein, non-starchy vegetables or a fruit, a small grain or starchy vegetable serving, and good fats such as olive oil and nuts. Balanced meals promote satisfaction and satiety.

Eat until you've had enough. Eat until you are about 70 percent full. If you are used to eating until you are uncomfortable, you may want to work on redefining your definition of how much is enough.

Enjoy your food! Savor your foods with your eyes and nose as well as your mouth. Letting all of your senses play a part can enhance your enjoyment and help you to feel more satisfied. Smell your food; notice the texture; enjoy the dance of the flavors on your tongue.

Do not eat in front of the TV or computer. Eat slowly and without distraction. It is hard to notice the body's cues while engaged in other activities. Try eating without the TV on, without reading emails, the newspaper or surfing the Internet.

Set the table. Set the table for yourself. Include music and candles to ramp up the ambience if this will help you to fill any void you may be experiencing.

Eat slowly. Enjoy slowing down and really intuitively getting in touch with your body. Chew your food completely. This helps the food digest and gives your body time to send necessary signals regarding fullness. Try chewing each bite at least 10–20 times. Take at least 20 minutes to enjoy your meal.

Eat mindfully at every possible meal. Write down what you learned about yourself while eating mindfully.

EXAMPLE

Mindful Messages: I found that I eat a lot more food and eat until I am uncomfortably full when I eat in front of the television. I also found that I enjoy my food when I listen to great music while I eat.

What did you learn?

_____
_____
_____
_____
_____
_____
_____

_____
_____
_____
_____
_____
_____
_____
_____
_____
_____
_____
_____
_____
_____
_____
_____
_____
_____
_____

STAY HYDRATED DURING THE CLEANSE PROGRAM

The Life-Affirming Power of Water

The secret elixir for cleansing our bodies is all around us. Water covers two-thirds of the planet, and yet most of us do not drink enough. And we should.

The liver must have adequate hydration to do its job. Dehydration lowers the liver's total productivity. Without proper hydration, the liver cannot metabolize fat as quickly or efficiently. If you allow yourself to become dehydrated, you are also setting yourself up to store fat.

During the first few days of drinking more water than your body is accustomed to, you will be running to the bathroom constantly. This is normal, and it will pass. Your body is flushing itself of the water it has been storing between cells and around fat cells. This process takes a while, but this is a beautiful thing happening to you. As you continue to give your body all the water it needs, it gets rid of the water it was holding on to in your ankles, your hips, and thighs, as well as around your belly.

Water is the best beauty treatment. It flushes out impurities in the skin, giving us a clear, glowing complexion. Water improves muscle tone; muscles that have all the water they need contract more easily, making workouts more effective.

How much water is enough?

Not that much. You should drink an ounce of water for every two pounds of body weight you carry. So if you are 160 pounds, you will want to drink a minimum of 80 ounces of water a day. Spread your water consumption throughout the day. Don't let yourself get thirsty. If you feel thirsty, you are already becoming dehydrated. Drink before you get thirsty. Water is in ample supply on The Cleanse Program.

Do you think water is yucky? Drinking other fluids will certainly help hydrate your body, but the extra calories, sugar, fake sweeteners, additives and whatever else are not what you need and can be harmful as well as counterproductive.

When you drink all the water you need, you will notice a decrease in your appetite, possibly even on the first day. If you are serious about becoming leaner and healthier, drinking water is an absolute must. While on The Cleanse Program, water is most definitely on the menu. You can add a slice of lemon, lime, grapefruit or even cucumber in your water to make it more flavorful.

STOP COUNTING SHEEP

Understanding the Sleep-Weight Connection

Sleep plays an incredibly important role in a healthy lifestyle. According to research conducted by the *National Health and Nutrition Examination Survey* (NHANES), people who receive less than eight hours of sleep each night are at a greater risk of being obese than their fully rested counterparts. Sleep deprivation leads to poor habits. When we are sleep deprived, we may crave comfort foods such as carbohydrates. When we are sleep deprived, the more we eat, the more we crave. Some people may not eat enough because eating can make us tired, which can lead to undernourishment. We often use stimulants to raise our energy level during the day, and then consume alcohol to fall asleep at night causing us to wake up between 2 am and 4 am. Waking up throughout the night will cause fatigue, a greater appetite and poor dietary choices the following day.

According to the NHANES study, participants who slept five hours per night 73 percent more likely to become obese than participants who experienced seven to nine hours of sleep each night. Participants who got only two to four hours of sleep per night were 87 percent more likely to become obese than people who slept a full seven to nine hours. And, participants who got six hours of sleep were 27 percent more likely to become obese than those who got seven to nine hours. Those who slept more than nine hours were 11 percent less likely to be obese or overweight.

How To Get Plenty Of ZZZs

Sleep is our time to repair and regenerate and getting seven to ten hours of high quality sleep is imperative for a healthy life. Even one night of little to no sleep can have an impact on the health of your bodily systems. Chronic sleep deprivation raises the body's cortisol levels (the stress hormone) and can even be a precursor to insulin resistance, which can result in the development of diabetes.

Many people rely on a late afternoon snack packed full of stimulants to get them through the second part of their day. What they may not realize is that stimulants may continue working long after its effects are desired. Even heavy meals and alcohol can prevent a good, quality night of sleep as can exercising or engaging in stimulating activities in the evening.

If you struggle to get a good, full night of sleep, there are some simple lifestyle changes you can make that will help you get the rest your body requires in order for you to achieve maximum health. Take this time during The Cleanse Program to honor your body's cry for sleep.

Action Tips

Have a challenging workout early in the day, rather than in the evening. Physical exercise helps with sleep because it burns off some of the tension, energy and stress that may be pent up.

- Try gentle yoga or stretching or even meditation in the evening.
- Take a hot bath infused with organic lavender essential oil.
- Read something that is soothing and entertaining rather than an intense novel or business book.
- Do not watch TV in bed or work on the laptop as these artificially stimulate the nervous system.
- Keep a notepad beside the bed and write your thoughts down at the end of the day so that you are able to end your day with a clear mind.
- Eat a light dinner.

- Set your alarm and get your body accustomed to going to bed and waking at a set time.

ENVIRONMENTAL TIPS

Check that your room is an appropriate cooler temperature. We tend to sleep better if the room is below 72 degrees. Studies show that 65-67 degrees is optimal.

Is your room dark enough? Put curtains or blinds in windows. You may need to wear an eye mask to shield any disruptive lighting caused from an outside source such as a street lamp. The body requires complete darkness in order to generate melatonin, which is the hormone associated with sleep. You should not be able to see past your outstretched hand in the dark.

SUGGESTED SUPPLEMENTS

B vitamins assist the body in making and using the chemicals necessary for a good night's sleep. Take a B vitamin early in the day and enjoy an additional energy boost throughout the day, as well as a deeper sleep at night. Both calcium and magnesium will calm your nervous system and should be taken about one hour before you are ready for bed. Both Melatonin and GABA are the brain's main inhibitory neurotransmitter and amino acid derived from proteins. Melatonin puts you to sleep and GABA assists the body in achieving a good quality sleep. GABA's action mechanism is what many of the prescription sleeping pills mimic. The amino acid Tryptophan and its derivative 5-HTP converts to serotonin, which then converts to melatonin for a good night sleep (Note: Do not take supplemental tryptophan or 5HTP if you are taking SSRI or anti-depressant drugs).

REV UP WITH REM

Quality sleep is essential to your health and to your detoxification process. A deep sleep should put your brain in a state of rapid eye movement (REM). REM is the state where most dreams, especially vivid dreams, occur. Most likely if you never get to that REM state, you probably never dream. So, if you are not dreaming, your body is most likely not receiving the regeneration necessary for optimal health. Ideally, you want to be in bed by 10 pm and wake up around 6 to 7 am. If you can get and stay on this schedule, you will find that you feel better.

If you are a person who goes to bed at 2 am and wakes up at 8 am chances are you feel like you have been run over by a Mack truck. If you can get to bed a little earlier and even wake up earlier, you will find that you feel more refreshed because you are actually going with the rhythm of the world. Most people feel better if they go to bed by 10 pm and wake up before 7 am. The quality of your sleep and the hormonal activities are improved when you go to bed earlier in the night.

We are able to condition ourselves to be "day people" or "night people" due to artificial light. There are no true night people. People who work shift work resulting in sleeping at odd hours have a higher risk of diabetes, high blood pressure and cardiovascular disease. By forcing yourself to stay up, you are reducing your quality of life. Quite honestly, without the artificial lighting that we have now, we would all go to sleep when it gets dark.

If you need assistance getting to bed early, you may want to try a relaxing exercise. Lie down and focus on relaxing your body. Start at your feet and begin relaxing each body part gradually moving up your body. Relax your feet, then your ankles, then your calves and then your knees and so on. Don't go to sleep at this point, but just get your body in a position where you can relax. Bring awareness to each body part. Relax and say goodnight to your body, and allow each muscle to relax and rest.

While on The Cleanse Program many people find that the sleep that was elusive is now easy to obtain. Even more often, people will find they sleep longer than 9–10 hours and that is okay. Your body is just recharging and restoring. It is not a sign of something amiss. Remember, sleep assists us in repairing from our day, rebalancing hormones, de-stressing, as well as assists in maintaining youthfulness. Sleep is not something we can bank—we lose the benefits each night we do not have deep sleep.

SUGGESTED BUT NOT REQUIRED SUPPLEMENTS

Why Use a Supplement to Cleanse?

Dietary cleanses are generally gentler than cleanses that require significant amounts of supplements. The Cleanse Program is primarily a dietary cleanse. Supplements are not required, and you will see and feel results even if you do not add any supplements. However, adding supplements to The Cleanse Program can make this process all that more effective and may also reduce your symptoms.

First, supplements cannot replace or override a crappy diet. Ingesting fish oil cannot undo eating a biggie, meaty, cheesy burger and fries every day. Supplements are exactly what the word means—nutrients, herbs and enzymes that supplement or boost your nutrient levels to improve different chemical reactions and activities of the body.

In my private practice at my wellness center, we do not use supplements, nutrients herbs and other products to help change chemical imbalances and improve body functions. Most of my clients have metabolic and nutritive testing through the Metabolic BluePrint℠ program (www.MetabolicBlueprint.com) that determines what supplements (based on individual lab results) are needed to balance the individual's body function. Unfortunately, I do not have the ability through this book to test you. So, all of the recommendations I am making in this section are generally safe for people to take and will gently influence detoxification activities and improve digestive function.

I believe it is unwise and unsafe to take supplements that are designed to alter liver detoxification or significantly impact kidney function without knowing a person's individual metabolic and chemical function. For this reason, I do not think liver cleansing with herbs is safe for everyone; therefore, I do not recommend embarking on those types of cleanses alone without testing and supervision. For some people, taking herbs without the knowledge of their individual body functions is much like opening pandora's box and can potentially make you sick.

The following supplements help cleanse the body without pushing the metabolic functions too quickly. You can order all of these supplements at www.CleanseTheBook.com.

- Cleanse Detox Formula (hypoallergenic detox powder with protein support)
- Detox Support: AdvaClear to improve detoxification in the liver
- Digestive Enzymes: Azeo-Pangen Extra Strength with meals to assist with digesting foods
- Stomach Acid Support: Metagest with meals containing proteins
- Omega-3s: EPA/DHA 720 Gel capsules
- Greens Powders: PhytoGanix Powdered Greens made from vegetables and fruits
- Glutamine powder: Glutagenics for amino acid and detoxification support

- Probotics: Ultra Flora Plus DF(dairy-free)
- Digestive herbs can be helpful for constipation but are often not necessary during the cleanse. If you have a tendency to be constipated, I often recommend Smooth Moves tea because it is mild and effective.
- Herbal Teas

Over the years, I have found that changing breakfast from a toxic white food-fest to something more nutrient-dense is the most difficult hurdle cleansers have to get over. The western world has become addicted to toast, bagels, cereal, pancakes, sugar, coffee and other foods that are not on The Cleanse Program westerners are averse to trying soups (eaten by millions of people in Asia each morning) and "dinner" foods for breakfast. For that reason, I have sourced the best meal replacement food that you can use to replace breakfast. It also works for snacks and other meals in a pinch.

UltraClear Renew is designed to help restore normal healthy detoxification and elimination functions. It is a comprehensive protein shake formula designed to softly support both phase I and II liver detoxification pathways while also providing antioxidants and protein. It is made of rice protein, the most hypoallergenic form of protein. I prefer rice protein to whey, egg or soy protein for obvious reasons—we are removing egg, soy and all dairy for the cleanse.

If you would like to order protein powders and supplements recommended for The Cleanse Program please visit www.CleanseTheBook.com.

THE POWER OF DIGESTIVE ENZYMES

Enzymes work as catalysts of biochemical reactions. Enzymes accelerate the speed of a chemical reaction (i.e., the chemical mixture it takes to break down foods). Enzymes are not destroyed or changed in the process. There are many types of enzymes, and each type does a specific function.

Foods contain enzymes, especially raw foods, fermented foods and sprouted foods. Enzymes can be supplemented as well with or without foods. The nice thing about enzymes is that if the particular molecule they work on is not present, the enzyme does nothing. For example, the enzyme lactase must come in contact with lactose, the sugar in dairy products that can cause gas and digestive complaints, in order to accomplish the chemical reaction of breaking down the lactose into glucose. No lactose, no action for the lactase to perform. Lactase just hangs out and moves through the digestive tract.

We have two types of enzymes in our bodies. There are metabolic or proteolytic enzymes and digestive enzymes. The digestive enzymes help break down the proteins in our food. Proteolytic enzymes are required for every chemical action that takes place inside the body.

Digestive enzymes transform food into energy for the body's use by breaking down complex proteins, fats and carbohydrates into smaller, simpler and more usable forms. Digestive enzymes act on the components in food to break it down. Without this transformation, digestion and assimilation of nutrients is difficult to impossible. Digestive enzymes should always be taken before or while eating to be effective.

Proteolytic enzyme supplements are anti-inflammatory, meaning that they assist the body in the healing efforts. Our immune systems use proteolytic enzymes to destroy invaders. When we supplement with proteolytic enzymes, our immune system's effectiveness is greatly increased. Proteolytic enzymes can also digest bacteria, fungi, molds and viruses that reside within the bloodstream. They will also act as a detoxifier, and because of this, may produce some symptoms of detoxification. If you have arthritis, chronic pain or stiffness, you may benefit from taking more enzymes between meals.

Dosing: Enzymes taken between meals (several hours away from food) break down accumulated toxins that contribute to inflammation or pain. These are proteolytic enzymes. Enzymes taken with meals improve digestion and aid in cleansing the digestive tract. These are digestive enzymes. Be sure to follow the dosing instructions on the bottle. Many enzymes work as both proteolytic and digestive enzymes—the only difference is when you take them.

FISH OIL AND OMEGA-3S

The fatty oil from fish and certain plant/nut oils contain omega-3 oils that reduce inflammation. Fish oil contains both docosahexaenoic acid (DHA) and eicosapentaenoic acid (EPA), while some nuts (English walnuts) and vegetable oils (canola, flaxseed/linseed, olive) contain alpha-linolenic acid (ALA).

ALA is known to be a source of energy for the body, and it is converted into DHA and EPA; albeit, to date we do not definitively know how efficient the body is at this conversion. Current research shows the body may only convert 5–10 percent of ALA to EPA and even less, only .01–5 percent, to DHA. So a person should not rely solely on ALA as a primary source of omega-3 fatty acids. Flax oil, which is on The Cleanse Program, is a source rich in ALA.

DHA, found in fish oil, is a long-chain fatty acid and is found in large concentrations in the brain, the eyes, the nervous system and heart. It plays an important role in the structural integrity of these parts of the body and is required for their proper functioning. DHA is required for proper brain function and development as well as for visual acuity and is the primary fatty acid in the brain and retina. Low levels of DHA in the blood have been shown to be related to low serotonin levels in the brain, which can affect mood. DHA is a key component in the central nervous system and also plays an important role in maintaining proper cardiovascular health.

EPA, the other main component in fish oil, is another important long-chain omega-3 fatty acid. However, unlike DHA, it is not stored as well in the body. So you must eat it on a regular and ongoing basis to maintain proper levels.

Similar to DHA, EPA plays a role in reducing the triglycerides and has mild blood thinning properties. EPA also moderates the immune response reducing chronic inflammation. It is thought that EPA plays less of a role in mood than DHA, but studies have not been conclusive.

Omega-3 fatty acids are important to the body. I consider a high-quality fish oil to be something that most people should integrate into their daily living. The benefits far outweigh any inconvenience or cost. I recommend that you research the fish oil that you use. The process used to remove methylmercury and PCBs (toxins) and refine the fish oil is expensive, and you want to be sure you are not getting contaminated fish oil. The old adage is true, "You get what you pay for." High quality fish oil is worth paying for. Visit www.CleanseTheBook.com to purchase fish oil specifically recommended for The Cleanse Program.

You will be consuming flax oil on the cleanse as food, so you will be getting ample ALA. Adding high quality fish oil will improve the benefits you experience on the cleanse. I recommend supplementing with 2000mg a day of fish oil. If you find that you "burp" fish oil, you can freeze the pills, or better yet, take it before you eat.

FABULOUS FIBER

Fiber is a form of carbohydrate that the human body is not able to digest for energy. As such, it passes through the human digestive tract undigested. Insoluble fiber, which is found in most kinds of vegetables and in psyllium husks, acts as a bulking agent and encourages the colon to move, flushing out old toxins that are released. If you are constipated, adding additional fiber with additional water will help you achieve more frequent bowel movements.

Soluble fiber is present in all plant foods, especially beans and other legumes, whole grains and certain fruits and vegetables. Root vegetables such as sweet potatoes and carrots are excellent sources of soluble fiber, and the skins contain insoluble fiber. Broccoli, bananas, apples and berries are also good sources of soluble fiber.

The short-chain fatty acids produced through the fermentation process created by gut bacteria of soluble fiber in the large intestine serve to stabilize blood glucose levels, lower (LDL) cholesterol in the blood, increase the production of immune cells and promote colon health. It has been shown that soluble fiber prevents the formation of intestinal inflammation and polyps, aids in the absorption of certain minerals and is a food source for the helpful bacteria in the colon.

The flax meal is high in soluble and non-soluble fiber. Apples are also high in pectin and other fiber, explaining the proverbial "An apple a day keeps the doctor away." Flax and apples are in ample use on The Cleanse Program.

GREEN POWDER SUPPLEMENTS

Vegetable greens are one of the most simple and mild ways to cleanse the inside of the body, helping to draw out toxins while supplying minerals, antioxidants and vitamins. Powdered greens are usually freeze-dried powders of the actual vegetables in high concentration; so you will get the equivalent of six servings of vegetables in one serving of green powders. Don't think you can skip your veggies and just do greens! It doesn't work like that. Powdered greens are your insurance policy. It just ensures you have more value in your diet. I prefer powdered greens over packaged and bottled juices because bottled juices are often pasteurized and/or contain preservatives, increasing acidity and robbing them of nutritional value. To order the Cleanse Green go to www.CleanseTheBook.com.

GLUTAMINE

Glutamine is a non-essential amino acid (building blocks of protein) found in the body. In fact, it is the most abundant free-form amino acid. It is non-essential because glutamine can be manufactured by the body to meet the physiological demands. However, there are times that glutamine becomes an essential amino acid (required by the diet) due to metabolic stress situations gastrointestinal damage, cancer or poor diet.

Under such conditions, additional intake of glutamine to meet the increased demand can be beneficial. Glutamine serves as a source of fuel for cells lining the intestines, and it's involved in more metabolic processes than any other amino acid. Glutamine can pass through the protective blood-brain barrier, and because of this, it is known as brain fuel. It is essential for maintaining amino acid balance in the body during times of severe stress. It is used by white blood cells and contributes to normal immune-system function. Glutamine also promotes the maintenance of a healthy digestive tract.

Glutamine can prevent the kind of muscle loss (wasting) that can accompany prolonged bed rest or illnesses such as cancer and AIDS. Stress and injury (including surgical trauma) can cause the muscles to release glutamine into the bloodstream. As a result, stress or illness can lead to the loss of skeletal muscle; therefore, one of the benefits of L glutamine is to prevent muscle loss (wasting).

The following foods are good sources of dietary glutamine: beef, fish, poultry, raw parsley, raw spinach as well as legumes.

Glutamine supplementation is considered safe when used with proper dosing guidelines. The most common side effects of glutamine supplementation include the following: constipation and bloating, which can be alleviated by drinking plenty of water. However, anyone with cirrhosis of the liver, kidney conditions, Reye's syndrome, or any type of disorder that can result in an accumulation of ammonia in the blood are advised to avoid supplemental glutamine. Pregnant and nursing women should only take an amino acid such as glutamine after consulting a physician.

While on The Cleanse Program, you can optionally take L-glutamine in your gut healing pudding. For most people, the recommended L-glutamine dosage is between 1000mg–3000mg daily for general health and repair of the intestinal lining. There are too many variables to give an exact amount for each individual, but let your body be your guide. Start out on the lower end, and if you feel you need to increase the amount just monitor how you feel. If you take a large daily dose and feel sick to your stomach, lower the dose.

PROBIOTICS

Probiotics are dietary supplements or foods that contain beneficial bacteria that are found naturally in the body. Although healthy people do not necessarily need to supplement with probiotics to be healthy, these microorganisms may provide some health benefits such as assisting with digestion and helping protect against harmful bacteria and supporting the existing colonies in the gut. In addition to supplements, probiotics can be found in such foods as Kiefir, kombucha, fermented foods, miso and cultured foods. There is a growing public and scientific opinion that probiotics taken as foods or supplements can help treat or prevent illness.

Probiotics may help the following:

- Treat digestive issues such as irritable bowel syndrome (IBS) and colitis.
- Shorten the duration of intestinal infections and treat diarrhea especially after antibiotic use.
- Prevent and treat inflammation following colon surgery (pouchitis).
- Prevent and treat vaginal yeast infections and urinary tract infections.
- Prevent eczema in children.

Some researchers believe probiotics may improve general health. A small 2005 study in Sweden, found that a group of employees who were given the probiotic Lactobacillus reuteri missed less work due to respiratory or gastrointestinal illness than did employees who were not given the probiotic.

The interesting thing is probiotics have been found to be beneficial in improving immune system function, treating digestive disorders such as Crohn's disease and ulcerative colitis. However, recent studies have shown that in order to maintain that effective boost, you must continue to take probiotics long-term.

Probiotic supplementation will allow the newly introduced probiotics via your supplement to vacation in your gut. Probiotics thus far have not proven to actually re-colonize the digestive tract. If you need probiotics for managing digestive complaints, you may want to stay on them long-term to experience lasting effects. Additionally, rotating brands and various combinations is also best to get a broad spectrum of coverage.

CLEANSING TEAS

Herbal teas have been used for millenia for medicinal purposes, especially in Chinese and Ayurvedic medicine. Most drugs are based on actions exhibited by herbal plants and teas. Herbal teas are also fabulous for taste and comfort.

Today there are many varieties of herbals teas, some of which are specifically recommended for use while on The Cleanse Program. The good news is that not only are they naturally caffeine free and healthy, but the tea consumption counts as part of the daily fluid intake requirement.

You may find you like one tea over another based on taste. They are all effective and some have different methods of action to assist in cleansing. You can buy herbal teas already prepared, or you can make your own. It is all a matter of preference and convenience.

I use the medicinal qualities of teas to mildly cleanse my system. Three of my favorite teas are ginger tea with lemon zest and juice, which I drink in the morning. I drink licorice root tea throughout the day and red clover tea at night. Any one of these teas will assist with cleansing. Getting a combination will also work synergistically to ramp up the cleansing process in a safe and enjoyable way—you get to relax while sipping tea.

Ginger and lemon tea serves as a diuretic. Lemon is good for stimulating digestion and even reducing calcium deposits in the kidneys. Ginger is great in soothing digestive woes. You can use the dried herb or fresh ginger. Just pour the boiling water over the herb and steep for a few minutes before adding lemon juice or zest.

Milk thistle tea is known to protect the liver and reduce inflammation of bile ducts resulting in decreased bile flow from the gall bladder. The key constituent of milk thistle is silymarin. Silymarin is the substance that enables milk thistle to give protection to the liver.

Dandelion root tea is one of the safest and most popular herbal remedies; it strengthens the liver and gallbladder by promoting the flow of bile, reducing inflammation of the bile duct and helping to get rid of gall stones. This is due to the active component taraxacin. Be careful if you have an active problem with irritable stomach or bowel, or if you have an acute inflammation.

Licorice root tea is often used to soothe an upset stomach and to treat stomach ulcers. It can help with heartburn and acid reflux. Licorice tea is said to have a calming effect and help alleviate stress. I have one caution for licorice tea: it can interfere with some medications and can cause increased blood pressure and shortness of breath in people suffering high blood pressure.

Fenugreek tea has active components of alkaloids, lysine and L-tryptophan. Fenugreek tea has the ability to aid the digestive process. It may help regulate blood sugar levels and may induce production of insulin, lower the bad cholesterol levels and can be used as an effective laxative. However, as with any herb, fenugreek should not be taken by pregnant women except when advised by a physician.

Burdock root tea has been used as a blood purifier, diuretic, catalyst for stimulating bile secretion and sweating, as well as to help skin conditions such as eczema, psoriasis and poison oak/poison ivy.

Lemongrass tea is great for reducing mucus, relieving headaches, balancing skin tone and is a mild sedative. The herb is used as an analgesic and is effective in reducing muscle pain. Lemongrass acts as a diuretic and eliminates excess water retention by promoting urination.

Lemon balm tea is a strong antibacterial and antiviral herb. It is calming to the nervous system and digestion in a tea form. A great combination when brewing lemon balm tea is to add a little bit of stevia to create a more desirable taste and to help your immune system if you are susceptible to seasonal allergies.

Chamomile tea is a great sleep inducer. It is also known for helping with colds and menstrual cramps.

Red clover tea is best used as a liver and blood purifier. Studies have shown it relaxes the nerves and treats coughs. It is also used to treat rheumatic or gout pain. Gargling with red clover tea can help sore throats since it acts as a mild sedative.

Rosehip tea is high in vitamin C and antioxidants and is a great herb to boost the immune system. If you feel you are coming down with a cold or get sniffles once you start the cleanse process, this is a good herb to introduce into your system.

However you decide to make your cleanse tea, whether store bought tea bags or by brewing your own with the actual herbs, teas are a convenient way to promote body functions and assist in the detoxification of your body.

SKIN CLEANSING

Because our skin is the largest organ of elimination, detoxification should include some type of skin cleansing. Some heavy metals can actually be released through the skin's pores when we sweat. It has been documented that our skin's sweat glands can perform as much detoxification as one, or both, kidney(s). Therefore, it is very important to support our skin for optimal detoxification. If our kidneys are damaged, helping the skin will indirectly but effectively help the kidneys.

Good skin care is vital to the health of our body. Anything that comes in contact with our skin has the potential to be absorbed and then transported through our blood stream to other areas of the body. Using chemical-laden skin care products is not wise, even though they are less expensive then organic products. These chemicals may be absorbed into our circulation and provide more toxins for our liver to process. For example, aluminum in deodorants has been implicated in breast cancer and Alzheimer's. We are not made out of cast iron, and even the chemicals in our soaps and shampoos will make a difference with our health.

Most people do not experience the ill effects of these subtle chemicals because their liver is able to metabolize them. Individuals who are environmentally toxic from other exposures often react to even the lowest levels of toxins in self-care products. Chemically toxic people will experience a great change in their health when using natural soaps and shampoos. Make a point to only use natural skin care products.

Cleansing our skin is rather simple. First, we need to bathe daily using natural soaps that do not contain toxins such as sodium laurel sulfate or parabens. Then we need to care for the skin by using only natural oils, lotions and organic or natural products. Even the clothes we wear can make a big difference in our health. Synthetic fibers do not absorb sweat (toxins), while natural fibers such as cotton will absorb toxins. Our clothes come in contact with our largest organ—the skin—if the clothes are toxic, your skin will absorb those toxins. So how can we improve skin detoxifications?

Sweat

First, sweat often, as in daily! Exercise that produces ample sweat not only helps us to stay lean, it helps us increase detoxification and remove the nasty stuff. Good sweaty exercise can be aerobic, warm yoga, working out outdoors in good weather or any other activity that works up a sweat. It does not matter how you get your sweat on, *just sweat*.

Sauna

Sauna baths, especially FAR-infrared saunas are great for removing toxins from the skin and regenerating one's health and energy. Saunas help to reduce physical stress by boosting circulation and triggering the production of endorphins—the "feel good" hormones. Besides these physiological effects, a sauna session also contributes to stress reduction simply by providing a peaceful and relaxing environment away from the stress of the day.

The traditional sauna has many health benefits such as relief from pain and muscle stiffness as well as relief from arthritis. Saunas also help in cleaning the skin. By taking in the steam from a traditional sauna, one can get a good relief from common complaints such as congestion, muscle and joint pain.

Generally, the traditional wood or the electric stove heats the air in the sauna much like an oven, but the infrared heaters provide heat using FAR infrared rays—the rays you feel when you are out in the sun on a sunny day. The infrared is a frequency band of light-wave that people cannot see. The heat produced is called Infrared Radiation (IR) or Far Infrared Radiation (FIR). These rays do not produce atomic radiation or sunburn, which is common with Ultraviolet Radiation. Humans emit Infrared Radiation and the IR from the sun is the cause of most of the Earth's heat. There is no risk to FAR infrared exposure. Infrared saunas do not produce steam, so in treating ailments such as breathing problems, they are not very useful. But they perform well in relieving arthritis pain and are an excellent source for working up a good sweat.

Compared to traditional saunas, infrared saunas have some advantages. For people who prefer cooler saunas, infrared saunas have the feature of heating up to low temperatures with the FAR waves penetrating the body at higher heat. This allows the individual to stay in the sauna for longer. This feature also makes FAR saunas cost effective because they use less electricity. With its advantage of operating at a lesser cost, IR saunas heat very quickly compared to the conventional saunas. FAR infrared saunas do not heat the air so the quality of the air is the same inside and outside.

Far Infrared Saunas have been shown to remove heavy metal toxins (including mercury), and fat-stored (lipophilic) toxins, plus metals trapped in connective tissue and the brain. They also increase the eliminative, detoxifying and cleansing capacity of the skin by stimulating the sweat glands. Each FAR infrared sauna session causes a brief, beneficial increase in body temperature.

Medical research shows that regular use of a FAR infrared sauna may be as effective for cardiovascular conditioning as exercise. As the body heats up, it cools itself by sending blood from the internal organs to the extremities and the skin, thus increasing heart rate, cardiac output and metabolic rate. In the 1980s,

NASA concluded that FAR infrared stimulation is the ideal way for astronauts to maintain cardiovascular conditioning during long space flights.

Toxins can play a significant role in preventing us from losing weight, as well as in causing us to gain weight. The body will even create fat to store chemical toxins when they exceed the body's ability to excrete them. Those who have been unsuccessful at dieting often have a toxicity problem and will find success after using a sauna to eliminate the chemicals stored in the fat cells that can impede weight loss. Those wishing to lose weight should also note that the cardiovascular effect from a single sauna session may burn as many as 500 calories.

By dilating blood vessels, infrared heat increases blood circulation to injured areas, speeding up the healing process and relieving pain. Infrared heat has also been used extensively in the treatment of arthritis, rheumatism and muscle spasms. Profuse perspiration deeply cleanses the skin, creating beautiful and improved tone, texture and color.

DRY SKIN BRUSHING OR WARM TOWEL RUBBING

Dry skin brushing helps in removing the outer dead skin layers and keeps the pores open. The brushing action will remove dead skin cells and open the pores to enable a freer flow of toxins. Another good method of skin brushing is with vigorous toweling off after bathing. Towel roughly until the skin is slightly red. Change towels often because the towel will contain toxins. Even better, you can use a washcloth (scratchy one) warmed with hot water and wrung out to rub in a circular motion increasing circulation and removing dead skin cells. I recommend doing this process at least once a day or in the morning and before bed.

To start, use a brush, warm washcloth or towel and vigorously rub in a circular motion starting at the feet and working your way up each leg. Then rub your arms from the hands up. Next rub the torso from the bottom all the way up to the clavicle bone above the heart on the left side of the body. Your lymphatic system dumps into the circulatory system right above the heart. Starting at the most distant parts of the body from the heart allows you to coax the lymphatic system to move toxins out of the body.

Detoxification Baths

Now that you know that your skin absorbs and excrete toxins, it probably makes sense that the right kind of bath can help remove toxins on top of being a great way to relax. The important thing to remember is that bubble baths usually contain harsh chemicals that you do not want to absorb. During The Cleanse Program, you will be using healthy additives to create the best cleansing baths.

Ingredients:

Combine the following in a standard bathtub:

- 1/2 cup of baking soda
- 1/2 to 1 cup of Epsom salt

If you have a garden tub, use 1.5 cups of your chosen ingredient. You may also add lavender for sleep or grapefruit or tangerine citrus essential oils to the water to sweeten the scent and improve detoxification.

Soak for 15–20 minutes, and then scrub the skin gently with soap on a natural fiber washcloth. This is also a great time to use your brush. Within a few minutes the water will turn murky and "dirty."

Enjoy a detoxification bath three times a week during The Cleanse Program and once a week for maintenance.

LYMPHATIC DRAIN THERAPY

At my wellness center we provide manual therapy to improve lymphatic drainage. Lymph Drainage Therapy (LDT) is an original hands-on method of lymphatic drainage developed by Bruno Chikly, MD, of France. Using anatomical science and distinctive manual processes, LDT enables practitioners to detect the specific rhythm, direction, depth and quality of the lymph flow anywhere in the body. From there the therapist use their hands to perform Manual Lymphatic Mapping (MLM) of the vessels to assess overall circulation and determine the best alternate pathways for draining body-fluid stagnations.

Therapists work with flat hands, using all the fingers to simulate gentle, specific wave-like movements. These subtle manual maneuvers activate lymph and interstitial fluid circulation as well as stimulate the functioning of the immune and parasympathetic nervous systems. It is shown that when these actions are accomplished, the results can be:

- Reduction in edemas (swelling) and lymphedemas of various origins
- Detoxification of the body
- Regeneration of tissue, including burns, wounds and wrinkles

- Anti-aging effects
- Relief of numerous chronic and subacute inflammations, including sinusitis, bronchitis and otitis
- Relief of chronic pain
- Reduction in the symptoms of chronic fatigue syndrome and fibromyalgia
- Anti-spastic actions to relieve conditions such as some forms of constipation
- Deep relaxation to aid insomnia, stress, loss of vitality and loss of memory
- Reduction of adiposis and cellulite tissue

To find a licensed Lymphatic Drain Therapist near you go to: www.upledger.com.

CLEANSING EXERCISE

If your lymphatic system is not blocked, rebounding is a good way to keep it moving. I often use rebounding between lymphatic drainage therapy to enhance the effects of the treatment. Rebounding exercise utilizes a mini trampoline to bounce the body up and down. Rebounding is an excellent activity for circulating lymphatic fluid. Something fascinating happens when you start moving up and down—you begin to subject your entire body to the forces of acceleration and deceleration, plus gravity. At the bottom of the bounce, your whole body comes to a gradual stop. Then, it increases in speed as you spring upward. The combination of vertical deceleration followed instantly by vertical acceleration of your entire body, combining with gravity, increases G-force, which is felt by every cell in your body. Our cells react to this environmental stimulation the same way they react to any other environmental change—they adjust and become individually stronger. The upward vertical action gives you a moment of weightlessness with no G-force.

Our cells depend upon a process called diffusion. Diffusion is the movement of fluid through the semi-permeable membranes. Diffusion helps to carry oxygen, nutrients, hormones and enzymes into the cell and also flushes out metabolic waste from the cell. The rate of diffusion of water into and out of the cells under normal conditions is 100 times the volume of fluid inside each cell each second. The alternation of the cells of your body between an increase in G-force and a no G-force increases the diffusion of water into each cell at least three-fold! Nothing beats that kind of cellular cleansing. Rebounding acts like a washing machine pulling fluids into the cells on the downward action and pulling toxins out of the cells on the upward action.

If a rebounder is not in the cards for you, elliptical trainers and snowshoe trainers work in a similar, but not quite as effective, way to move the lymphatic system.

10
Domestic Detox

> *Treat the Earth well. It was not given to you by your parents. It was loaned to you by your children.*
> *– Kenyan Proverb*

KYM GLASS, TESTIMONIAL

I achieved great success with The Cleanse Program. I found the program to be so educational. Betty Murray made the entire process fun and easy. I wasn't sure what to expect during The Cleanse Program. I was just hoping I would feel better. During the 21-day detox, I lost three inches in my waist and four pounds. I feel much better, and I have more energy than ever before. The information I obtained about how toxins affect our everyday life has been amazing to hear. I was surprised I did not lose more weight; however, losing that many inches off my waist in three weeks was amazing!

I decided to remain on a revised eating plan since finishing The Cleanse Program. I am keeping a lot of the great foods in my day-to-day regimen and as of my twenty-eighth day (at the time of writing this), I have lost an additional inch in my waist.

Did you know the home environment is often more toxic than an urban city? As a matter of fact, according to the Environmental Protection Agency, indoor pollution can be five to ten times more toxic than outdoor pollution and is typically contaminated by as many 20 to 150 different toxins in concentrations of 10 to 40 times of those outdoors.

Everything our bodies consume impacts our toxicity levels. It is much easier to be cognizant of your fluid and food consumption than it is the air you breathe and the surfaces you touch on a daily basis. Because we absorb toxins through our skin, we are in a near constant state of toxic contact. When you consider the carpet you stand and sit on, the fibers and detergents that are in your clothing and the cleaning agents you use to "sanitize" your home, you can quickly ascertain the seriousness of the toxicity that may exist in your home.

If you are using traditional cleaners within your home, you may be surprised to find that the actual cleaning agents may be just as harmful, if not more, than the bacteria and soil you are attempting to wipe away. Conventional cleaning products are made from a vast array of surprisingly toxic chemicals. When using the chemicals within the home, they can actually remain suspended in the air for hours and even days as you and your family inhale them and absorb them through skin to surface contact. Even more alarming, when chemicals from various products come in contact with one another, they can combine to create a different, and possibly more toxic chemical.

Unfortunately, product-labeling regulations do not require the manufacturer to warn the consumer of the hazardous materials contained within the product. Household cleaners are the only household products regulated by the Consumer Product Safety Commission under the Federal Hazardous Substances Labeling Act, but the manufacturers are not required to reveal their ingredients, as these are considered to be trade secrets. Sadly, government regulations are designed to protect the proprietary information of the corporation at the expense of the consumer's health, as well as the health of the environment. Certain words such as "danger," "warning," or "caution" certainly alert the consumer that the product is not safe for human consumption, but these words provide very little information regarding the seriousness of the unknown substances and no information at all regarding the seriousness of long-term exposure.

One of the first steps in understanding how to put your home through a detox is to understand the terminology of the household cleaning industry. When it comes to understanding household chemicals, understanding the distinction between natural, organic and synthetic is crucial. All matter in the universe is composed of a combination of the approximately 110 atoms, or elements. There are ninety-two elements that occur naturally and one of those is carbon. Carbon is a unique element that is associated with all living things. Chemical compounds containing carbon are referred to as "organic chemical."

In the nineteenth century, scientists began compounding naturally occurring carbon with manmade chemicals and continued to refer to these compounds as organic chemicals; however, an important distinction is that these manmade compounds are actually "synthetic organic chemicals" versus the truly organic, "natural organic chemicals." Throughout the years and through a multitude of scientific research and experimentation over 85,000 chemicals are now available and widely used throughout a multitude of consumer products. According to the Breast Cancer Fund, complete toxicological screening data is available for only 7 percent of these chemicals, and more than 90 percent have never been tested for any side effects on human health. So, of the 85,000–100,000 known chemicals currently being utilized in consumer products, only 5,595 have data indicating their effect on human health. In 1995, the National Toxicological Program concluded from various tests results that an approximate five 5–10 percent (4,250 to 8,500) of all chemicals in production could be expected to be carcinogenic in the human body. The majority of the chemicals have yet to be regulated, much less even recognized by the United States government.

All of these 85,000 chemicals at some point find their way into the air, water, land and ultimately into the human body. These chemicals may eventually produce an effect known as "acute toxicity," which is defined as an immediate and negative health crisis. What is more alarming, however, is the chronic toxicity that these chemicals produce in our bodies. Chronic toxicity manifests itself in a multitude of chronic health disorders. The symptoms of chronic toxicity appear over time and can include asthma, allergies, cancer, endocrine, immune and nervous system damages, reproductive and developmental disorders, organ damage, as well as the general condition known as multiple environmental chemical sensitivity (MCS) or environmental illness. MCS is a body-wide allergic reaction to repeated contact with toxic chemicals.

THE GOOD NEWS

The good news is that there are many truly natural and organic cleaning products on the market that are effective in terms of cleaning the home, as well as safe for your family. You want to purchase products that are produced with biodegradable chemicals. Biodegradability means that the product can be recycled by nature, or that the chemicals can be broken down into their natural parts through the actions of microorganisms. Biodegradability also implies that the chemical will not accumulate in the environment. When a chemical does not biodegrade, it continues to become more and more concentrated, and thereby increases in toxicity with time. Because a toxic agent increases with time, a relatively benign chemical can become highly toxic over time as it continues to build up within the body or the environment.

There are many wonderful products that can greatly assist in cleaning out the toxins in your home, and by using these products you can also cut back on the residual toxicity. Seventh Generation, Mrs. Meyers and Shaklee are just a few brands currently on the market that are making great strides in detoxifying household cleaning. While it is true that we are what we eat, perhaps a more accurate statement is that *we are what we ingest, breathe and touch.*

GET GREEN & GET CLEAN

Did you know your houseplants do more than keep your home beautiful? They also keep your home clean. Plants take in carbon dioxide and create oxygen, and they also protect against pollution. The following plants can remove domestic toxicity, as well as suppress the growth bacteria spores and mold within your home, which ultimately keeps your household air cleaner and safer for you and your family.

- Dracanea removes trichloroethylene, which is found in paints, adhesives and dry cleaning solvents.
- The Snake plant removes formaldehyde, which is commonly found in ceiling tiles, flooring, fabrics and even cosmetics.
- The Moth Orchid removes xylene and toluene both of which are emitted by ceiling tiles, caulk, flooring and computer screens.
- The Peace Lily removes benzene, which is found in plastics, paint, synthetic fiber and even detergents.
- The Areca Palm removes just about all domestic toxins. This is a great plant to have in multiple rooms throughout the house.

THE PROBLEM WITH PLASTIC

Plastics contain chemicals that are endocrine disruptors. An endocrine disruptor is a synthetic chemical that when absorbed into the body either mimics or blocks hormones disrupting the body's normal functions. This disruption can happen through several ways: altering normal hormone levels, halting or stimulating the production of hormones, or changing the path the hormones travel through the body. All of this disruption results in altering the functions that these hormones control.

Studies have found that endocrine disruptors can leach out of plastics, including the type of plastic used in water bottles, food storage and plastic wrap. Many endocrine disruptors stay active in the environment causing long-term pollution. And that is not all. These pollutants accumulate in fat—*your fat!*

Do you want proof that endocrine disruption really exists? According to a study headed up by scientist Patricia Hunt at the Case Western Reserve University in Cleveland, Hunt's team discovered unusual genetic defects in the eggs of laboratory mice. She traced it to their hard plastic cages, which were apparently out gassing small amounts of BPA into the mice's environment.

The team claims that its research has shown that even the very smallest traces—20 parts per billion in drinking water—can alter 8 percent of eggs. Under normal circumstances only 1 percent of eggs are usually defective. Humans are exposed to similar BPA levels through exposure to plastics in bottles, food storage, liners of canned goods and other plastic usage. Now, as we all know, multiple studies have shown that BPA is dangerous.

So do you think that this is the first time that the safety of plastic has been questioned? Think again! Earlier studies implied that exposing animal fetuses in the womb to levels of BPA similar to those found in the environment can have a detrimental effect on sperm count and testicular development. However, other studies—some commissioned by the plastics industry—have found BPA to be completely safe.

BPA is an endocrine disrupter that mimics the hormone estrogen, the hormone most associated with breast and ovarian cancer. Studies have shown harmful effects on animals using as low as 2–5 parts per billion. Many canned foods have plastic liners with BPA levels well over that range.

Hunt's groups showed that BPA might also harm the human ovarian egg's DNA; this damage might be inherited by the offspring formed from those eggs. It seems that BPA stops chromosomes from dividing up equally before egg cells divide, possibly by interfering with estrogens' normal activity. That estrogenic effect is especially taxing to our already potentially overburdened estrogen balance.

What plastics should you watch out for? Let's start with the latest bad for you plastic-nista Bisphenol-A (BPA). BPA is mainly found in polycarbonate plastic, which is labeled with the number seven. It is often used in plastic food wrap and in the resins that coat the inside of metal cans for food. It is so ubiquitous in today's products that it is even in refrigerator shelving, water bottles, plastic food storage containers, water pipes and flooring.

A study by the U.S. Center for Disease Control found that about 93 percent of the population in the U.S. have BPA in their body at a mean concentration of 2.7 parts per billion. In studies, animals given BPA well under the U.S. maximum limit have been observed to display hyperactivity (hmm ... ADD/ADHD), insulin resistance (type II diabetes?) at 10 ppb/day, early puberty at 2.4 ppb/day, and other types of harm to sex organs even at levels of approximately 0.025 ppb/day, which is much lower than what was in more than half of the people in the CDC study.

Bisphenol-A could also be making us fatter. In a recent study, researchers at the University of Missouri-Columbia fed quantities of BPA to mice during their early development to produce traceable amounts in their bodies that were lower than levels found in most people by the CDC study. Guess what? The mice became significantly fatter as adults than their fellow mice that were not given BPA.

Unfortunately, there are many other endocrine disruptors similar to BPA. Educate yourself and limit your exposure. (Much of the information: code & symbol, name, properties, product applications can be found on the Web sites of plastics industry organizations [SPI, APC and CPIA]).

Recycling Number 1

Polyethylene Terephthalate (PET or PETE). This type of plastic is found in plastic soft drink and water bottles, beer bottles, mouthwash bottles, peanut butter and salad dressing containers, oven-proof plastic bags, oven-proof pre-prepared food trays. These plastics potentially leach the chemical "antimony trioxide." Antimony trioxide is a catalyst regularly used in the production of PET plastic resin. Exposure to antimony trioxide for extended periods of time has shown signs of chronic toxicity, including respiratory tract and skin irritation. This toxin passes into breast milk as well as into the placenta. Exposed females that work with the chemical have exhibited an above average incidence of menstrual problems and of late-term miscarriages and delayed development in their children during the first year.

Recycling Number 2

High Density Polyethylene (HDPE) is found in milk, water, juice, cosmetic, shampoo, dish and laundry detergent bottles, trash and retail bags, yogurt and margarine tubs and cereal box liners. Research is ongoing on this type of plastic. This type of plastic is believed to be safer than many of the others.

Recycling Number 3

Polyvinyl Chloride (V or Vinyl or PVC) is found in toys, clear food and nonfood packaging, shampoo bottles, medical tubing, wire and cable insulation, film and sheet. It is also found in construction products such as pipes, fittings, siding, flooring, carpet backing and window frames. The active plasticizers are the phthalates Di(2-ethylhexyl) phthalate (DEHP) and butyl benzyl phthalate (BBzP). DEHP and BBzP are endocrine disruptors mimicking the female hormone estrogen. These have been linked to asthma and allergic symptoms in children. Also, according to some medical studies, the plasticizers added to PVC may cause certain types of cancer (cholangiocarcinoma, angiosarcoma, brain cancer).

Recycling Number 4

Low Density Polyethylene (LDPE) is used in plastic as a barrier to moisture, increased toughness, flexibility and ease of sealing. It can be found in bread and frozen food bags and squeezable bottles (i.e., ketchup and mustard). Research is ongoing as to the effects LDPE has on the human body. This type of plastic is thought to be safer than many of the others.

Recycling Number 5

Polypropylene (PP) is known for its strength, resistance to chemicals, resistance to heat, ability to withstand moisture, versatility and resistance to grease and oil. It is found in ketchup bottles, yogurt containers and margarine tubs, and in medicine bottles. Research is ongoing into Polypropylene's long-term effects. This type of plastic is thought to be safer than many of the others.

Recycling Number 6

Polystyrene (PS) is a versatile plasticizer used for insulation and clarity. Polystyrene is also easily "foamed" (Styrofoam). It is used in compact disc cases, foodservice applications, grocery store meat trays, egg cartons, aspirin bottles, cups, plates and cutlery. Styrene migrates from polystyrene containers into the container's contents, especially when oily foods are heated in such containers.

Styrene is an endocrine disruptor mimicking the female hormone estrogen, and much like other endocrine disruptors, it has the potential to cause serious reproductive and developmental problems.

Recycling Number 7

The number seven is a "catchall" indicating the product in question is made with a resin other than the above six, or is made of more than one resin used in combination. Usually the seven category includes polycarbonate, acrylonitrile styrene (AS), styrene acrylonitrile (SAN), acrylonitrile. Dependent on the combination of resins, styrene (ABS), nylon or acrylic, the plastic will have increased strength, rigidity, toughness and temperature and chemical resistance.

AS/SAN is used in mixing bowls, thermos casing, dishes, cutlery, coffee filters, toothbrushes, outer covers (printers, calculators, lamps) and battery housing. The incorporation of butadiene during the manufacture of AS/SAN, produces ABS, which makes it an even tougher plastic. ABS is used in LEGO toys, pipes, golf club heads, automotive parts and protective headgear.

Plastic has become so ubiquitous in our "throw everything away" society that there is no way to remove it completely, and plastics do provide some very important functions. For example the health care industry would not be able to have sanitary equipment and tubes without the use of plastic.

We can, however, reduce our use of unnecessary plastics in our lives and have a greater impact on our detoxification and body systems.

The following simple changes can have very beneficial results: Change out food storage for leftovers to Pyrex or glass storage instead of plastic. Use glass drinking glasses and pitchers instead of plastic. Reduce eating fast foods and disposable foods. Install water filtration systems in your home to reduce bottled water consumption.

DO-IT-YOURSELF GREEN CLEANING RECIPES

General Cleaning Agents

- Baking soda (sodium bicarbonate) is an all-purpose, nontoxic cleaner perfect for general cleaning, deodorizing and removing stains, as well as softening fabrics.

- Borax (sodium borate) is a natural mineral that kills mold and bacteria. Borax

is a great alternative to bleach as it deodorizes, removes stains and boosts the cleaning power of soap.
- Castile and vegetable oil based soaps clean just about everything.
- Cornstarch is perfect for starching clothes. It will also absorb oil and grease.
- Use herbs and essential oils for disinfecting and as an all-purpose home fragrance.
- Lemon juice cuts through grease and removes perspiration and other stains from clothing—use as a bleach alternative.
- Use salt (sodium chloride) when you need an abrasive cleaning agent.
- Use all natural toothpaste when you need a mild abrasive.
- Vinegar (acetic acid) cuts grease, removes stains and is an excellent water softener.

Air Fresheners

- Place cloves, cinnamon sticks, allspice or other favorite spices in a pot of water, and simmer for one to two hours.
- Simmer orange or lemon rinds in a pot of water for several hours.
- Place baking soda in an open container and sprinkle several drops of your favorite essential oil for scenting. Place in any area that may require odor absorption.
- Place several pieces of white bread in the refrigerator to absorb odor.

All-Purpose Cleaners

- Mix vinegar and salt together for a good surface cleaner.
- Dissolve four tablespoons baking soda in one quart of warm water for a general cleaner.
- Sprinkle baking soda on a damp sponge and use to clean and deodorize all kitchen and bathroom surfaces.
- Combine liquid Castile soap and baking soda with water to clean the floors, walls, counters, tubs and sinks, cat boxes and anything that can be well rinsed.
- Create a paste with baking soda, salt, vinegar and water.

Disinfectants

- Mix one-half cup of borax into one gallon of hot water or undiluted vinegar.
- Mix one-half cup of borax into one gallon of hot water, and add a few sprigs of fresh thyme, rosemary or lavender. Steep for 10 minutes, strain and cool. You may choose to add essential oils in place of the fresh herbs. Store in a spray bottle.
- Combine two tablespoons borax, one-fourth cup lemon juice, and two cups hot water. Combine the borax and lemon juice with the water in a spray bottle. Use as you would any commercial all-purpose cleaner.
- Isopropyl alcohol is an excellent disinfectant. Sponge on to the surface and let dry. Use in a well ventilated area and wear gloves.

Glass Cleaners

Each of the following can be used in a spray bottle:

- Straight, undiluted vinegar
- Equal parts vinegar and water
- The juice of one lemon mixed with two cups of water
- One-half cup vinegar or lemon juice, two cups of water, one-fourth teaspoon vegetable oil based soap (such as Murphy's Oil Soap)

Scouring Powders

- Use a non-chlorine scouring powder such as Bon Ami.
- Baking soda or dry table salt are both mild abrasives that can be used as an alternative to chlorine scouring powders. Simply put either baking soda or salt on a sponge or onto the surface, scour and rinse.

Non-Abrasive Soft Scrubber

Combine one-fourth cup borax, vegetable oil-based liquid soap (such as Murphy's Oil Soap) and one-half teaspoon lemon oil in a bowl. Mix the borax with enough soap to form a creamy paste. Add the soap and blend well. Scoop a small amount of the mixture onto a sponge, wash the surface, and then rinse well.

Toilet Bowl Cleaners

- Baking soda and Vinegar Cleaner: Sprinkle baking soda into the bowl and then spray the vinegar into the bowl. Scour with a toilet brush.
- Borax and Lemon Juice Cleaner: Mix enough borax and lemon juice to form a paste and cover the stain. Flush toilet to wet the sides and then rub the paste onto the stain. Let the mixture sit for two hours and then scrub thoroughly. For less stubborn stains, sprinkle baking soda around the rim and scrub with a toilet brush.
- Borax-Vinegar Cleaner: Flush the toilet to wet the sides of the bowl. Sprinkle borax around the toilet bowl and then spray with vinegar. Leave the mixture on for several hours or overnight before scrubbing with a toilet brush.
- Soap & Baking Soda Cleaner: Mix liquid Castile soap and baking soda or borax together, and then scrub with a toilet brush.

Drain Cleaner

For slow drains, use this drain cleaner once a week to keep drains fresh and clog-free.

- One-half cup baking soda
- One cup white vinegar
- One gallon boiling water
- One-half lemon
- Pour baking soda down the drain and/or disposal and follow it with the vinegar. Allow the mixture to foam for several minutes before flushing the drain with boiling water.

Tub and Tile Cleaners

- Baking Soda: Sprinkle baking soda onto the surface and rub with a damp sponge. Rinse thoroughly.
- Vinegar and Baking Soda: To remove film buildup on bathtubs, apply vinegar full-strength to a sponge and wipe. Next, sprinkle baking soda on the surface and rub with a damp sponge. Rinse thoroughly with clean water.
- Vinegar: Vinegar removes most dirt without scrubbing and will not leave a film.

Use one-fourth cup (or more) vinegar to one gallon of water.

- Baking Soda: To clean grout, combine three cups of baking soda into a medium-sized bowl and add one cup of warm water. Mix into a smooth paste and scrub into grout with a sponge or toothbrush. Rinse thoroughly and dispose of leftover paste when finished.
- Rub the area to be cleaned with half a lemon dipped in borax. Rinse well, and dry with soft cloth.

Porcelain Cleaner

Cream of Tartar: To clean porcelain surfaces, rub with cream of tartar sprinkled on a damp cloth.

Plumbing Fixtures

- To clean stainless steel, chrome, fiberglass, ceramic, porcelain or enamel fixtures, dissolve two tablespoons of baking soda into one quart of water. Wipe onto the fixtures and then rinse.
- Vinegar & Paper Towels: Cover hard lime deposits around the faucets with vinegar-soaked paper towels. Leave the paper towels on for about one hour before cleaning. This will leave the chrome clean and shiny.

Oven Cleaners

- The first step is prevention. Keep a sheet of aluminum foil on the floor of the oven, underneath but not touching the heating element.
- Clean up the spills as soon as they occur.
- When spills occur and while the oven is still warm, sprinkle salt or baking soda on the spill. If the spill is completely dry, wet the spill lightly before sprinkling on salt. When the oven cools, scrape away the spill and wash the area clean.
- Sprinkle water on the oven bottom and cover with baking soda. Let this sit overnight. Wipe off and apply liquid soap with scouring pad and then rinse.
- Prevent grease buildup in your oven by dampening your cleaning rag in vinegar and water before wiping out your oven.
- Sprinkle or spray water followed by a layer of baking soda. Rub gently with a very fine steel wool pad for tough spots. Wipe off the scum with dry paper

towels or sponge. Rinse well and wipe dry.

- Mix two tablespoons of vegetable oil-based liquid soap and two tablespoons borax in a spray bottle. Fill the bottle with hot water and shake well. Spray on the oven and leave for 20 minutes. Scrub off.

Refrigerators

- To clean exterior and interior walls, dissolve two tablespoons baking soda in one quart warm water and wipe all surfaces. For stubborn spots, rub with baking soda paste. Be sure to rinse with a clean, wet cloth. (This works well on other enamel-finished appliances as well.)
- To clean interior fixtures, such as vegetable bins and shelves, wash in hot soapy water, rinse well and dry.

Fragrant Kitchen Rinse

Use any of the following essential oils, alone or in a combination. Add four drops of oil to each pint of water. Pour into a spray bottle, store in a cool, dark place. Use as a final rinse after cleaning kitchen surfaces.

- Eucalyptus
- Pine
- Lavender
- Cypress
- Lemon
- Lemongrass
- Lime
- Thyme
- Grapefruit
- Orange
- Wintergreen
- Rosemary
- Sage

Pots and Pans

- Soak or boil a solution of two tablespoons of baking soda per one quart of water in each burned pan. Let stand until particles are loosened, and then wash as usual. Use a mild or moderate abrasive if necessary.
- To clean a greasy pan easily, add one or two teaspoons of baking soda to the water in which it is soaking.

Copper Pan Cleaner

Sprinkle surface of pans with coarse salt. Rub salt into stains with the cut half of a fresh lemon.

No-Stick Cookware

To remove stains from non-stick surfaces, pour a solution of one cup water, two tablespoons of baking soda into a pan and simmer five to ten minutes. Do not allow mixture to boil or to boil over the side of the pan. Wash in hot soapy water, rinse and dry. Apply a light coating of cooking oil.

Enamel, Ceramic or Glass Baking Dishes

Soak in hot soapy water, then scour with salt or baking soda and rinse thoroughly.

Dishes

- Use liquid or powdered soap in lieu of a petroleum-based detergent. In dishwashers, use equal parts borax and washing soda.
- Use baking soda and liquid soap.

Drinking Glasses

Occasionally soak drinking glasses in a solution of vinegar and water to get them really clean. When a quick dip for crystal glassware is needed, prepare a solution of baking soda in tepid-cool water (one level teaspoon to one quart) and brush with a soft toothbrush. This is a great solution for glass coffee makers and thermoses.

Spot-free Dishwasher Rinse

Add one cup of white vinegar to the rinse compartment of your automatic dishwasher. Wash dishes as usual.

Coffee/Tea Stains

Rub baking soda on cups or counters with coffee stains.

Drain Opener and Garbage Disposal Cleaner

Use this drain cleaner once a week to keep drains fresh and clog-free.

- One-half to one cup baking soda

- One cup white vinegar
- One gallon boiling water
- One-half of a lemon
- Pour baking soda down drain/disposal, followed by vinegar. Allow the mixture to foam for several minutes before flushing the drain with boiling water.

Garbage Disposal

Grind ice and used lemon and/or orange rinds until pulverized to eliminate garbage disposal odors while cleaning and sharpening blades.

Carpets/Upholstery

- General Carpet Stain Remover: A great nontoxic carpet stain remover is club soda. Soak spot immediately with soda and blot until the stain is gone.
- Pet Urine on Carpet: Dab area with a towel to absorb as much as possible, wash spot with liquid dish detergent, and rinse with one-half cup vinegar diluted in one quart of warm water. Lay towels or paper towels over the spot and weight down to absorb excess moisture. Let stand for four to six hours, then remove toweling, brush up nap and let dry completely. Use an electric fan to speed drying.
- Red Wine Stain Remover: Red wine stains can be removed from carpet by rubbing baking soda in and vacuuming.
- Baking Soda Grease Remover: To remove grease spots from carpets, first sop up the liquid with a sponge, and then rub a liberal amount of baking soda into the spot. Let it absorb overnight. Remove the excess and vacuum the area.
- Cornstarch Grease Remover: To remove grease spots from carpets, first absorb excess with a sponge, and then rub a liberal amount of cornstarch into the spot. Let the cornstarch sit overnight and then vacuum.

Carpet Freshener:

- 4 cups baking soda or cornstarch
- 35 drops Eucalyptus essential oil
- 30 drops Lavender essential oil
- 25 drops Rosewood essential oil or any combination of essential oils

Measure 4 cups of baking soda into a bowl and add essential oils. Break up any clumps that form, stir until well mixed. Sprinkle powder mixture, and let it sit on the carpet for about 15 minutes then vacuum.

Herbal Carpet Freshener:

- 1 cup baking soda
- One-half cup lavender flowers

Crush the lavender flowers to release their scent. Mix well with baking soda and sprinkle liberally on carpets. Let the mixture sit for about 30 minutes and then vacuum.

Natural Rug Deodorizer:

- Sprinkle baking soda on carpets before vacuuming for a natural rug deodorizer.

Furniture Polish and Scratch Covers

This furniture polish should to be made fresh each time you use it.

- One lemon
- One teaspoon olive oil
- One teaspoon water
- Extract the juice from the lemon. Mix with oil and water. Apply a thin coat on your wood surface and let it sit for five minutes. Use a soft cloth to buff to a deep shine.

Floor Cleaners

- Use a pencil eraser to remove heel marks from the floor.
- For greasy, no-wax floors mix the following:
- One cup vinegar
- One-fourth cup washing soda
- One tablespoon vegetable oil-based liquid soap
- Two gallons hot water
- Combine all ingredients, and stir well to dissolve the washing soda. Mop as usual.

Silver Metal Cleaner

- Use toothpaste instead of a toxic silver cleaner to clean and brighten even your best silver. Use an old soft bristled toothbrush and warm water.
- Rub with a paste of baking soda and water.
- To magnetize tarnish away, soak silver in salted water in an aluminum container; then wipe clean.
- Soak in boiling water, baking soda, salt and a piece of aluminum foil.
- When a quick dip for silverware is needed, prepare a solution of baking soda in tepid-cool water and brush with a soft toothbrush.

Brass Metal Cleaner

- Mix equal parts salt and flour with a little vinegar and then rub.

Chrome Metal Cleaner

- Rub with undiluted vinegar.

Copper Metal Cleaner

- Rub with lemon juice and salt, or hot vinegar and salt.

Stainless Steel Metal Cleaner

- Rub with a paste of baking soda and water.

AUTOMOTIVE CLEANERS AND CARE

Windshield Wiper Frost Free Fluid

This vinegar and water combination will keep windshields ice and frost-free. Mix three parts vinegar to one part water. Coat the car windows with the solution.

Car Soap

Mix one-fourth cup vegetable oil-based liquid soap and hot water in a bucket. Wash your car on the lawn instead of your driveway to reduce runoff to the street or storm sewer.

Car Wax

- One cup linseed oil
- Four tablespoons of carnauba wax (available at automotive stores)
- Two tablespoons of beeswax
- One-half cup vinegar
- Put ingredients in the top half of a double boiler or saucepan. Heat the mixture slowly until the wax has melted. Stir, and pour into a heat resistant container. After the wax has solidified, rub it on the car with a lint-free cloth. Saturate a corner of a cotton rag with vinegar and polish the wax to a deep shine.

INSECTS & PESTS

Fleas and Ticks

Wash pets with Castile soap and water and dry thoroughly. Apply an herbal rinse made by adding one-half cup fresh or dried rosemary to a quart of boiling water (steep for 20 minutes, strain and cool). Spray or sponge onto pet's hair or fur, and massage into skin. Let air dry, do not towel dry as this removes the residue of the rosemary.

Roaches

- Mix equal parts boric acid with flour, and sprinkle around cracks and crevices.
- Mix equal parts boric acid with sugar, and sprinkle around cracks and crevices.
- Mix equal parts boric acid with cornmeal, and sprinkle around cracks and crevices.
- Diatomaceous earth (pure silica): sprinkle around flours, cracks and crevices.
- Set cucumber peels out on countertops overnight to repel roaches.
- Mix borax with a little brown sugar and flour, and sprinkle behind appliances, under sink and in corners. Cockroaches will carry the mixture back to their nests.

CAUTION: Boric acid and borax can be toxic to small children and pets, keep well out of their reach and inform other household members of the whereabouts and purpose of the borax and boric acid dough and/or powders. Always refer to safety precautions on the package.

Flies

Mix the following ingredients into a bowl and leave out in infested area.

- Two cups lavender flowers
- One cup rosemary
- One cup southernwood
- One-half cup spearmint
- One-half cup santolina
- One-fourth cup pennyroyal
- One-fourth cup tansy
- One-fourth cup mugwort
- One-fourth cup cedarwood chips
- Ten yellow tulips
- Three tablespoons orris root

Moths

Mix cedar chips, shredded newspapers and lavender flowers and scatter in the infested area. Moths do not like the smell.

CAUTION: Boric acid and borax can be toxic to children and pets, keep well out of their reach and inform other household members of the whereabouts and purpose of the borax and boric acid dough and/or powders. Ammonia should also be used with caution. Always refer to safety information and precautions on the package.

11
The Dietary Cleanse

> *Take care of your body. It's the only place you have to live.* - Jim Rohn

GETTING STARTED

If you chose to skip the Quick Start Guide, you will find all the detailed rules of The Cleanse Program in this chapter. If you dove right into your cleanse at the start of the book, you will find some repeated information in this chapter as well as more detailed information. Please take the time to get prepared before starting. Preparation will make all of the difference in the world. Lack of planning is where most people trip up when implementing new healthy habits. Give yourself every opportunity for success by planning ahead and preparing for The Cleanse Program. I have included a three-day preparation guide that you can use, or you may way to create your own plan that works with your lifestyle.

TALK TO YOUR DOCTOR

Please make your doctor aware any time you make changes to your diet or lifestyle. If you suffer from any illness, it is important that your doctor approves or is aware of any shifts in diet, lifestyle or exercise. Think of your relationship with your physician as a partnership, and that partnership works best when each party is honest and clear with one another. Informing your doctor of the details of your cleanse will be beneficial in the proper monitoring of your health. So, please disclose your plans. I am not promising your doctor will like hearing the word "cleanse" or "detox," and rightfully so. There are many drastic and downright dangerous detox programs, especially for individuals with compromised health situations. So your doctor's alarm with the word "detox" is justified. However, The Cleanse Program is gentle on the body and will reduce, not cause, stress.

You may be fortunate to have a doctor who advises on diet and lifestyle. Unfortunately, that is usually not the case. Doctors only get a few hours of nutrition education in medical school. Consequently, they are not usually well equipped to answer questions about nutrition. Some doctors may be less than approving when you say the word "detox." Feel free to share the book or the quick start guide with your doctor to ensure him/her that this is a very safe and healthy program.

If your doctor is concerned about The Cleanse Program, you can highlight the fact that The Cleanse Program contains real whole foods and healthy new eating habits. You will not be on any calorie restrictions on this program. You will be required to remove processed, toxic and fake "frankenfoods" such as hydrogenated oils, soda and fast foods from your diet.

SETTING GOALS

I always tell my clients that it is as important to identify why you want to do something, as it easier to do something when we are very clear with the "why." When we know the "why," we are more motivated to keep on our new path to wellness when challenges arise. And challenges will arise. So, let's find out why you really want to do a detox. Set aside some quiet time and answer these questions.

- What things do I need to begin doing to make my cleanse effective?
- What things do I need to stop doing to support myself in my cleanse?
- What areas of my life need support from others to make the cleanse succeed?
- What goals do I have for the cleanse?
- Do I want to lose some weight or lose inches in my mid-section?
  - If so, how much weight or how many inches?
- Do I want to see if foods are contributing to my feeling of dis-ease?
- Do I have fears about my risk for disease; if so, what are they?
- What are my feelings about a permanent lifestyle change?

I know it sounds like a business meeting when we start talking about goals, but I cannot tell you how important setting realistic and measurable goals is to your success on The Cleanse Program. In my practice, we use is a Tanita bioimpedance scale to measure body weight, fat pounds, lean muscle pounds, body fat percent and hydration levels before and after The Cleanse Program. We also get body measurements. "Cleansers" are typically very excited to get on the scale at the end to actually see the positive shifts they have created in their bodies.

Fat loss and weight loss are secondary goals of The Cleanse Program. The primary goals are to feel better, gain energy, improve negative health symptoms and obtain better sleep.

Take a few minutes to get clear with yourself. What are your measurable goals? Write your goals on paper or in your journal. You may want to post your goals in a place that allows you to see them every day. I post my cleanse goals on the inside of my bathroom wall cabinet, so I see them several times a day.

Here are some examples:

- I want to be sleeping through the night
- I want to get off the coffee/sugar rollercoaster
- To determine if changing my diet might reduce the symptoms of allergies, high blood pressure, diabetes, eczema, psoriasis, etc.
- To use The Cleanse Program to jumpstart my healthy lifestyle.

Now you write your own.

_____
_____
_____
_____
_____
_____
_____
_____
_____
_____
_____
_____
_____
_____
_____
_____
_____
_____

GET SUPPORT

It would be lovely if you only had to be concerned with yourself during The Cleanse Program, but most of us do not have the luxury of focusing exclusively on ourselves for three weeks. We have families, jobs, friends and other responsibilities that interact with us on a daily basis. Anyone who has ever dieted or tried to change their lifestyle will tell you that other people often unwittingly try to sabotage it. People may try and get you to go to for coffee or happy hour. Or, just have this one piece of birthday cake—it can't hurt you that much!

Friends, co-workers and family are not out to intentionally sabotage you. When people are presented with someone who is making significant changes in their life, it can cause fear for the other person. They may fear that you will not be interested in doing the same things. People may fear you will no longer want to be with them when you change. More often, their fears are a reflection of their own insecurities about their unmet desires or wants and how they may not be taking steps to make those things happen. It is important that your family, significant other and supportive close friends know that you are on The Cleanse Program. It is even more important that you let them know how important the program is to you. Tell them how they can help you during the cleanse process. People, for the most part, are interested in be helpful. Let them help you! They just need you to tell them how.

I have created some questions to help you start a script to use with family and friends in order to gain their support. Go through the following four questions, and ask yourself the same four questions for each potential challenge you may have regarding starting, staying on and succeeding on The Cleanse Program. Please do not skip this step, as it truly will help you.

Based on previous experience, what has been a challenge that has prevented you from successfully implementing a healthy change in diet? For example: Do you have problems being "good" at night after work when you have tried changing your diet in the past?

- What resources do you need to help you overcome this challenge?
- Who can you ask for support to help you?
- What specific steps can you take to ensure success in this area of your life?

Complete the following:

Dear _____,

I have started a Cleanse Program that will require me to change my lifestyle and habits for several weeks. I know that in the past I have struggled with _____
_____
_____
_____
_____
_____(question 1). I need your support to keep me in track in these areas: _____
_____
_____
_____
_____
_____
_____
_____ (question 2). I have asked you to do this because _____
_____
_____
_____
_____ (why you chose the person from question 3). These are the specific changes I will be making: _____
_____
_____
_____
_____
_____
_____
_____
_____
_____
_____

PREPARE YOUR KITCHEN

Get your kitchen ready! If you cannot find your kitchen because of the sea of mail that has taken over the counter or the kid's backpacks and art has taken up residence, it is time to get a little organization going. Save yourself time and frustration by creating a prep space that is easy to use. If the task looks too daunting, there are people that can help you get organized. Check out the National Association of Professional Organizers at www.napo.com.

You will not need any fancy kitchen gadgets such as juicers or a spiral slicer. A blender and a Crockpot are good items to have, but not required. A sharp set of kitchen knives, a cutting board and stainless steel pots or pans will be sufficient for you to do The Cleanse Program. A blender will be needed for the Cleanse Advanced recipes.

COOKWARE

The type of cookware you use is very important. Implementing ceramic-coated cast iron or stainless steel cookware can help you make great improvements with regard to the level of toxins you ingest and metals you absorb. Pyrex glass is also safe to cook with—just let it cool completely before washing to reduce the chance of it shattering.

Toxic Cookware

The following cookware is not on The Cleanse Program and should be removed from your kitchen entirely: anodized, Teflon and all "non-stick' surface cookware. With only a few minutes on a conventional stovetop, cookware coated with Teflon and other non-stick surfaces can exceed temperatures at which the coating breaks apart and emits toxic particles into the air. DuPont studies show at 680°F Teflon pans release at least six toxic gases, including TFE (tetrafluoroethylene), TFA (trifluoroacetic acid), HFP (hexafluoropropene), OFCB (octafluorocyclobutane), carbonyl fluoride, CF4 (carbon tetrafluoride), trifluoroacetic acid fluoride, perfluorobutane, SiF4 (silicon tetrafluoride), PFIB (perfluoroisobutane), HF (hydrofluoric acid), and particulate matter. At least four of these gases are extremely toxic. For example, PFIB is a chemical warfare agent, and MFA (monofluoroacetic aid) can kill people at low doses. HF is a highly corrosive gas.

Enough said! Teflon and anodized non-stick pans are bad news! Even though aluminum is not considered to be a heavy metal, it can be toxic in excessive amounts and even in small amounts if it is deposited in the tissues. Aluminum toxicity can cause symptoms of colic, rickets, gastrointestinal problems, interference with the metabolism of calcium, extreme nervousness, anemia, headaches, decreased liver and kidney function, memory loss, speech problems, softening of the bones and aching muscles. Many of the symptoms of aluminum toxicity mimic those of Alzheimer's disease and osteoporosis. Cooking with aluminum pans increases your exposure, especially if you cook acidic foods such as tomato sauces. By the way, municipal water is the largest source of aluminum in our diet.

PREPARE THE PANTRY

One of the most supportive things you can do is to get rid of the enemy! If your pantry, desk drawer at work or refrigerator is full of toxic, processed foods and junk, it will only make it harder to stay on The Cleanse Program. Some people reading this just got a vivid picture of mutiny in the house! What will the rest of the family eat? Well, they could participate with you on the cleanse with you. The Cleanse for Beginners is healthy for people of all ages, or you can simply remove the things that are most tempting to you.

When deciding what to toss and what to keep, a good rule of thumb is take a look at the food in question and ask yourself, "Does this remotely resemble anything found in nature?" If the answer is no, that piece of food is not on The Cleanse Program. Just in case you are not following me, here are some examples. The last time you drove by a farm, did see any wheat bread growing on stalks? I bet not! Did you see Special K flakes growing on vines? Absolutely not. They may say "whole grain," but they are not whole grains. Know that these are processed foods, period.

Remember this marketing rule: The amount of marketing, celebrity endorsements and advertising spent on a product is inversely proportional to the nutritive value of the product. What this means is soda pop, chips and other junk food require extensive advertising because they have no real food value.

Grains: That Means "WHOLE GRAINS"

Most grains are off limits during The Cleanse Program. Now is a good time to get rid of all of the processed grains hiding in the pantry. How can you tell if they are processed? Just read the section above again. The only grains that are whole grains are grains that are completely unprocessed: brown rice, basmati rice, millet, quinoa, amaranth, wild rice and many others. These are really seeds and should look like seeds. Anything that has been processed – flaked, baked, powered, floured, milled or hulled is off limits during The Cleanse Program.

Spices, Sauces and Marinades

Did you know that your spices, sauces and marinades contain some of the most toxic chemicals in food processing such as monosodium glutamate (MSG); texturized vegetable protein (TVP), which contains MSG; high fructose corn syrup and sodium benzoate. While on The Cleanse Program, you will be making your own salad dressings. I promise it is the easiest thing to do! So easy, in fact, that you will stop buying the toxin-laden dressings sold in stores.

Canned Goods

Canned goods should be your last resort vegetable option. Remember, fresh is best, frozen in a pinch and canned as a last resort. Canned foods are basically cooked to death. Many of the important nutrients such as vitamin C, minerals, sodium, calcium and potassium are diminished during the canning process. However, some foods do benefit from the canning process. For example, the nutritive value of the lycopene found in tomatoes actually increases during the canning process.

Canned goods are often lined with PBC-laden plastic (which you already know is bad) or tin. Tin, while not a heavy metal is still damaging to the body in excessive amounts. Tin has been found to irritate the gastrointestinal tract, cause headaches, bloating, diarrhea, nausea and vomiting.

Limit your intake of canned goods during and after the cleanse to a last resort food. I would rather someone choose canned green beans over skipping a vegetable because they did not have fresh or frozen on hand, but I do not recommend using them daily as your primary source of vegetables.

I keep canned legumes such as garbanzo beans and aduki beans on hand because of the long soaking and cooking times of beans. I also keep canned stewed and diced tomatoes as well as tomato sauce on hand for desperate times, but I only use them in a serious pinch.

Get With the Program

If you have not taken the Toxicity Assessment, go back to Chapter One and do it now. The assessment is designed to help you determine how aggressively you will do The Cleanse Program. Now, I know all the "type A" people (that would also be me) may want to go to the advanced recipes to step up the cleanse activities, even if it is their first time. It is up to you.

If you are a regular restaurant and fast food junkie, you may want to ease into The Cleanse Program. The Cleanse Recipes range from the Basic Cleanser to the Advanced Cleanser to assist those of you who swing pretty far on the junk food pendulum. Even without the advanced recipes, The Cleanse Program will provide great benefits to a "health nut" person as well as provide wonderful benefits to a cleanse newbee.

The Cleanse Program is designed to be 21-day program because that is how long it takes us to start to develop new habits. The body requires several weeks of detoxing in order to reduce inflammation, improve immune function and start shedding toxins. If you are sensitive to the most allergenic foods that have been removed from the diet during The Cleanse Program, it may take several weeks for the immune system to calm down and for you to feel the effects. After 21 days, you should be in the mode of developing new habits, and your body will be responding positively to your new changes. You could, and many of my Cleansers do, continue the program for a longer time if you find significant shifts in your health and well-being.

WHAT TO EAT

The Cleanse Program is a whole foods based detoxification. The following information provides everything you need to know about what foods to eat and how to prepare your selected foods.

Protein

Protein, including animal protein, is a necessary component of your body function and is required to assist in detoxification, building of new cells and even in your neurochemistry. You must have ample protein broken down into amino acids to assist in detoxing your body. However, living in Texas and seeing the portion sizes of what we serve in restaurants, I feel I must also say that you can get too much. Portions should not be over 8-ounces at a single meal even for the most strapping of men. Too much protein puts a significant burden on digestion and will cause a significant insulin response even if there is low carbohydrate consumption at the same time.

When shopping for protein choices from animal, fowl and fish, choose free-range, cage-free, grass fed and no hormone added sources whenever possible. Did you know that grass-raised, never grain-fed beef has a significantly lower level of fat, especially pro-inflammatory omega-6 fats and contains almost as much omega-3 fat as a wild caught piece of salmon? Grass-fed, free-range is the best possible choice for eating healthy protein.

Wild caught, especially cold water, fish are excellent choices for nutrient-dense proteins that are also high in omega-3 fatty acids. Avoid farmed raised fish when possible as they carry large amounts of industrial toxins and mercury in their meat. Grocery stores such as Whole Foods, Fresh Fields, Central Market and other health food stores often check their suppliers closely and can assure you a healthier choice of fish. Limit your fish intake to two to three times per week. Additionally, smaller fish such as sardines are a fabulous choice and have less of a chance of being contaminated with toxins because of their short lifespan.

Organic, free-range meats may occasionally be more expensive than conventionally raised meats. So, here are a few money saving ideas: First, think of meats, fish and fowl as a smaller portion of the plate. Also, many small local farms may not have organic certification because of the cost of certification but still provide high quality choices at often better than specialty grocery store prices. As an added bonus, we reduce our carbon footprint and improve the environment when we shop locally. For information about local farms in your area check out www.EatWild.com and www.WestonAPrice.org.

Protein Powders

While I am a proponent of whole foods nutrition, unadulterated protein powders, especially those designed with additional enzymes and amino acid profiles, are very beneficial for detoxifying the liver. Protein powders are also a way to have quick easy nutrition for an on-the-go lifestyle. Do not be swayed into going to mass-market smoothie shops though. They have hidden sugar and processing that you do not want to be ingesting.

There are a lot of protein powders on the market, many of which are not very healthy. Rice protein is the best protein powder choice for a detox as it is the most hypoallergenic of the protein powders. Hemp and pea protein are the next best choices.

It is important to use protein that is not denatured or heat processed. The heating or fractionating process damages the protein and making it appear foreign to the body. Protein powders were born out of the bodybuilding industry and many of the commercial powders contain fat burners, fractionated proteins and other additives. Stay away from these. The Cleanse Detox Formula is a rice protein that contains macronutrients to fuel detoxification pathways, a full multivitamin/mineral for detoxification enzyme support, and high levels of antioxidant support for safe detoxification.

Fat

Fats are the most misunderstood, misreported and misinterpreted foods. The lipid hypothesis assumed that there is a direct relationship between the amount of saturated fat and cholesterol in the diet and the incidence of coronary heart disease. The lipid hypothesis was proposed by a researcher by the name of Ancel Keys in the late 1950s. Interestingly enough, numerous subsequent peer-reviewed studies have questioned his conclusions but received little notice from the media.

Most people are surprised to learn that there is, in fact, very little evidence to support that a diet low in fat actually reduces heart disease or in any way increases one's lifespan. In fact, before 1920 coronary heart disease was rare in the United States. From 1910 to 1970, the proportion of saturated fat in the American diet declined from 83 percent to 62 percent. During the same period of time, the percentage of dietary vegetable oils in the form of margarine, shortening and refined oils increased about 400 percent while the consumption of sugar and processed foods increased about 60 percent. During the next 40 years, however, the incidence of coronary heart disease rose dramatically to be leading cause of death among Americans. If heart disease results from the eating saturated fats, you would expect to find a corresponding increase in saturated fat consumption in the American diet. The numbers just do not add up.

So what fats are really healthy?

Omega-3 fats or fish oils are good fats. Omega-3 fatty acids are essential fatty acids, meaning that they are essential to human health but cannot be made by the body. They have to be obtained through food. Omega-3 fatty acids can be found in fish, such as salmon, tuna, and halibut. Other sources for omega-3 fats are algae, krill, nut oils and some plants.

It is important to maintain an appropriate balance of omega-3 and omega-6 in the diet, as these two substances work together to promote health. Omega-3 fatty acids are anti-inflammatory and most omega-6 fatty acids pro-inflammation. Too much omega-6 fatty acids compared to not enough omega-3 fatty acids promotes the development of disease, while a proper balance helps maintain, and may even improve, health.

A healthy diet should have a ratio of one omega-3 fatty acid to three omega-6 fatty acids. The typical American diet tends to contain 14–25 times more omega-6 fatty acids than omega-3 fatty acids. Research reveals that this imbalance might be the significant factor in the rising rate of inflammatory disorders such as heart disease in the United States.

But what about those important the omega-6 oils?

Omega-6 fats are also essential and work in concert with omega-3 fats to balance body functions. For instance, omega-6 fat raises blood pressure, while omega-3 fat lowers blood pressure. Additionally, omega-6 fat promotes blood clotting while omega-3 fat hinders clot formation. Since they have opposing effects, the balance of these essential fats in the diet is imperative to your health.

Throughout human history, we have evolved on a diet that provided balanced amounts of these two fats. Over the last 100 years, our diets have changed dramatically, more so than it did for the first 250,000 years. First, food science made it possible to mass produce vegetable oils cheaply, and our variety of fats changed to one major source in foods—omega 6, with little to no omega 3 fats. Then, farmers began feeding livestock grains instead of their natural food choice of grass, which made the animals fatter (marbling) as well as higher in saturated and omega-6 fats. In addition, omega 6 fats, much like omega-3 fats, are fragile and can easily become rancid, which is very bad for your body.

The Standard American Diet is heavily comprised of pro-inflammatory omega-6 fats. We can reduce omega-6 fats by eliminating corn, safflower, soy and grapeseed oils, as these are already in abundance in our processed foods. However, it is important not to go overboard in trying to reduce too much omega-6 fat intake either. Too much omega-6 is not healthy and neither is too little—the goal is to achieve a balance of omega-3 and omega-6 fats.

MONO-A-MONO (MONOUNSATURATED FATS)

Monounsaturated fats or omega-9 fats are often referred to as "good" or "healthy" fats because they can lower LDL cholesterol and have been shown to have an anti-inflammatory effect on the body. Monounsaturated fat is found in avocados, almonds and other nuts and seeds. Omega-9 is not technically an essential fatty acid because the body can produce a limited amount, provided the essential fatty acids omega-3 and omega-6 are present. Studies show that monounsaturated fats lower cholesterol levels, thereby reducing the risk of cardiovascular disease as well as reducing atherosclerosis (hardening of the arteries). Omega-9 fats also play a role in reducing insulin resistance, thereby improving glucose (blood sugar) maintenance.

To include more monounsaturated fats, try sprinkling a few nuts or sesame seeds on a salad or over cooked vegetables; or use olive, walnut or avocado oil either in low heat cooking or sprinkle over your food after cooking. Do not use these oils in high heat cooking.

Saturated fats from animal and vegetable sources provide a concentrated source of energy in the diet; they also provide the building blocks for cell membranes and a variety of hormones and hormone-like substances. Studies now show that the right amount of saturated fats in our diet are not the cause of our modern diseases.

Saturated fatty acids constitute at least 50% of the cell membranes. They are what gives our cells integrity. They play a vital role in the health of our bones. For calcium to be effectively incorporated into the skeletal structure, a portion of the dietary fats should be saturated.

Saturated fats are needed for the proper absorption of essential fatty acids. Elongated omega-3 fatty acids are better retained in the tissues when the diet is rich in saturated fats.

Short-chain and medium-chain saturated fatty acids have important antimicrobial properties. They protect us against harmful microorganisms in the digestive tract.

What about Cholesterol?

Our blood vessels can become damaged in a number of ways—through inflammation caused by free radicals or because they are structurally weak or from infections. Cholesterol repairs the damage.

Cholesterol is required for your body to make vitamin D, a very important fat-soluble vitamin needed for healthy bones and nervous system, proper growth, mineral metabolism, muscle tone, insulin production, reproduction and immune system function.

So what kind of saturated fats should you eat?

Tropical Oils are more saturated than other vegetable oils. Coconut oil is one of my favorites. Coconut oil is 92% saturated with over two-thirds of the saturated fat in the form of medium-chain triglycerides. Coconut oil contains lauric acid. This fatty acid has strong antifungal and antimicrobial properties. Acquaint yourself with the merits of coconut oil for baking fats or occasional frying. Finally, use good quality butter as it contains butyric acid which also performs anti-bacterial activities.

VEGETABLES

Vegetables, especially green leafy vegetables, are severely lacking in most Americans' diets. Vegetables provide the body with much-needed vitamins, minerals, antioxidants such as vitamin C complex, various carotenes, and large amounts of alkaline-forming compounds that help us to maintain a proper systemic pH. Without these nutrients, the body slows down its chemical processes, increases stress and aging, and increases the likelihood for disease.

On The Cleanse Program, non-starchy vegetables are considered your primary food source and should be eaten liberally. I recommend that you use this time to investigate the section of the grocery store that you may be avoiding. Vegetables can and do taste good. You just have to experiment with your preparation techniques.

What are the most beneficial veggies? First, let me tell you that America's top "vegetables" (as considered by the American Dietetics Association) are corn and ketchup. These are not vegetables! Corn is a grain, and ketchup is sugar and vinegar with tomato added as coloring. Think about eating from a rainbow of choices—red, green, yellow, orange and so forth. A few examples of non-starchy vegetables include: (see next page)

- Asparagus
- Bell peppers (red, yellow, green)
- Broccoli
- Brussels sprouts
- Cucumber
- Kale
- Kohlrabi
- Lettuce
- Mustard greens
- Onions
- Dandelion greens
- Parsley
- Spinach
- Tomatoes
- Turnip greens
- Watercress

The majority of the body's minerals come from the vegetables you eat. For example, iron is found in dark leafy greens and in beets. Leafy vegetables are rich in chlorophyll, a substance that plants use to produce energy from sunlight. Chlorophyll's structure is very similar to hemoglobin, the molecule in our blood that carries oxygen to all the cells. The only difference is that hemoglobin contains an atom of iron in the center, while chlorophyll contains an atom of magnesium. This difference causes chlorophyll to be green while hemoglobin is red. Here are some other tasty tidbits of reasons to make friends with the vegetable kingdom!

- Leafy green vegetables are rich in magnesium.
- The radish, onion and cabbage families are excellent sources of sulfur, another important trace mineral.
- Sea vegetables such as kelp, dulse and Irish moss contain an extremely wide variety of trace minerals from the sea.
- Sea vegetables are extremely rich sources of minerals.

After digestion, vegetables and fruits have an alkaline residue, while almost everything else has an acid residue. To keep the body in a desirable acid/alkaline balance, you want to strive to consume about twice as much alkaline-forming foods as acid-forming foods (by weight). In other words, you must consume about twice as much produce as all other foods combined. So you want to think about vegetables being one half of your plate and the other food groups occupying the rest of the plate.

High Fiber Starchy Vegetables

High fiber starchy vegetables are vegetables such as peas, lima beans, red potatoes, yams and sweet potatoes, lentils, peas such as garbanzo beans and split peas. These foods contain vitamins such as Vitamin A, C and minerals such as potassium, selenium, germanium and calcium.

Generally, your diet should contain between 25 and 40 grams of fiber per day, and that 20–30 percent of the total fiber intake be soluble fiber. Most people have a much lower fiber intake than is recommended. The American average is about eight grams a day! Researchers who study the diets of our prehistoric ancestors say that they ate upwards of 100 grams of fiber per day; so we probably can handle very high amounts of fiber without difficulty.

Can't I Just Take Pills?

While fiber supplements can be helpful additions to a high-quality nutritious diet, and will be used during The Cleanse Program, supplements should never stand in for high quality nutrient-dense foods. There is some evidence that suggests simply taking pure fiber as a pill, or sprinkling high fiber additions over your food, does not carry all the same benefits as when it is actually in real food. Also, grain-based fiber additives such as wheat bran contain phytates that block the absorption of some nutrients.

If you are unused to eating a lot of fiber, increase the amounts gradually to prevent intestinal distress. You must drink a lot of water when taking fiber supplements or eating high-fiber foods, as all fiber absorbs at least some water. Fiber can, in rare cases, cause constipation if eaten without sufficient fluid.

Since large amounts of fiber can reduce absorption of some medications, it is best to take medication either an hour before, or two hours after, the fiber consumption. Many non-starchy vegetables provide a better quality and higher quantity of fiber than whole grains.

Grains

Yes, grains are also a source of dietary fiber. However, as you have already read, I am not a huge fan of a grain-based diet. Humans only started consuming grain in the last 10,000 years. Homo sapiens have existed for over 300,000 years. We know that modern-man existed on the planet for at least 70,000 years prior to ever eating grains. For 60,000 of those years, man was a gatherer and hunter eating mostly root vegetables, leafy greens and other vegetables and wild game.

Many people have a hard time digesting, assimilating and processing grains. As you know now, grains, especially those most ingrained in our culinary lexicon, are often sources of unknown allergies and sensitivities leading to malabsorption, weightgain, autoimmune disease, mood disorders and other problems. So, grains are not my favorite source of fiber, nutrients or carbohydrates. The vitamin and mineral profile of fruits and vegetables far exceed the profile of grain for providing nutrients needed by humans.

Grains are specifically the seeds from different types of grasses. Try searching for pictures of wheat, rice, oats, and even corn plants on the Internet, and you will notice they look similar to the grass that grows tall in unkept lawns and fields. There are a few grains that do not contain the peptide gliadin (gluten free) that have high fiber content and are allowed in small quantities on The Cleanse Program. Millet, quinoa and amaranth are allowed. You are probably wondering if I am recommending that you eat bird food. Yes, I am. These grains are often components found in bird food. However, these grains have fantastic nutrient profiles and are gluten-free.

If you want to eat grains on The Cleanse Program, you may have one serving of the following grains per day: brown rice, wild rice, basmati, forbidden rice, quinoa, amaranth and millet. These grains are usually sold in the bulk section or next to the bag rice and pastas.

Fruits

The glycemic index of a particular food, including fruit, is not as important as researchers once thought, if the food if is rich in nutrients and fiber. The fiber in whole fruits is much more important in blood sugar control than the glycemic index. Fiber rich fruits such as berries, apples, and pears are my favorite choices for The Cleanse Program as they provide a high level of antioxidants, vitamin C and nutrients to the body.

The berry family is rich in Vitamins A, C, E and beta-carotene as well as rich in the minerals potassium, manganese and magnesium. They are very high in fiber and low in sodium. All berries contain health-protecting antioxidants, compounds that prevent cancer-causing cell damage and may limit age-related diseases. Generally, the darker the berry color, the greater the antioxidant value. So blueberries, acai berries and goji berries are some of the best fruits for cleansing; however, all berries are good for you.

Antioxidants help to stop the production of free radicals. Free radicals are groups of atoms that impair the cells and the immune system, which leads to disease. Antioxidants bind the free electrons in free radicals so they can be neutralized and eliminated.

Anthocyanins create the darker hue in blueberries and other berries. Anthocyanins are antioxidants, known to reduce heart disease and cancer in humans.

Chlorogenic acid, another antioxidant, may slow the release of sugar into the bloodstream after a meal and help fight damaging free radicals.

Ellagic acid also appears to bind cancer-causing body chemicals, rendering them inactive. Raspberries have more ellagic acid than most other berries.

Catechins, the active antioxidant in green tea, seems to diminish the formation of plaque in the arteries, may suppress cancerous tumors and cell proliferation, and improves metabolic function.

Resveratrol is a substance that is produced by several plants but is in abundance in berries. It has a number of beneficial health effects, such as anti-cancer, anti-viral, neuro-protective, anti-aging, and anti-inflammatory effects.

So as you can see, fruit, especially berries, can be used to help your body detoxify. The best way of doing this is to use fruits as snacks and in a morning protein smoothie. Acidic tasting fruits, especially red grapefruits, lemons and limes have very strong detoxifying effects. A time-tested Auyrvedic remedy is to drink a glass of warm water filled with the juice of half a lemon to stimulate digestion, provide vitamin C to the liver for detxofication support and flush the lymphatic system. We will be using lemons and limes in filtered water throughout the day to help the body detoxify. Just make sure to brush your teeth or rinse your mouth out with plain water after drinking lemon or lime infused water as the acids can slowly breakdown the enamel on your teeth.

Lastly, apples are a great self-contained snack food that has body benefiting nutrients that will help you detoxify. Apples are a good source of vitamin C, vitamin A, biotin, folic acid, calcium, phosphorus, potassium and dietary fiber. The soluble fiber in apples is called pectin. Pectin helps to clear out the dangerous heavy metals such as lead and aluminum that we all pick up from our city air, food and water.

We want to rid the body of heavy metals, so the apple is important! Heavy metals can seriously interfere with your body's metabolic functioning. For example, mercury tends to suppress the levels of white blood cells in the immune system. Cadmium displaces zinc.

Unlike cellulose, another form of fiber, pectin is water-soluble; and therefore it does not affect fecal bulking. Pectin may also help eliminate bile acids from the intestines, thus short-circuiting the development of colon cancer and gallstones. It is useful as a natural chelating (binding) agent, which is why it is so good at mopping up unwanted heavy metals such as aluminum from the tissues for elimination from the body.

The nutritional value of apples will vary slightly depending on the variety and size of the apple. When eaten, it stimulates the secretion of digestive juices. Apples also contain natural substances that help prevent digestive and liver troubles.

WATER

Water—you need it, and you need the right amount of it. Relatively active adults need one ounce of water for every two pounds of body weight per day. Highly active adults need even more. An easy way to determine if you are getting enough water is by the color of your urine. If it is very pale or clear, you are well hydrated. If it is darker, you need to drink more.

Now that we have established how much water to drink, what about what kind of water? Mountain Valley water offers spring water for delivery to your home and office. And they will bottle your water in glass rather than plastic if you so desire. You can use large containers and fill safe, smaller, reusable BPA-free or stainless steel container from your delivered water; or you can also use a filter system, which is obviously a more substantial investment long term.

What about tap water?

On the positive side tap water is cheap, basically safe and is easily available. It has a neutral or slightly alkaline pH, and usually contains some good minerals and depending on where you live can have a good or a bad taste. Tap water and water filtration of infectious elements is one of the most significant health initiatives to increase human longevity on the planet. So, I am not knocking all it has done.

However, our municipal filtration systems are local and the quality of that filtration is dependent on what is in the ground water, the quality of the equipment and the amount of money funneled into improvements. One city might have state of the art filtration; another city might have a system 100 years old. Tap water can be polluted with many industrial chemicals that are not totally removed by the water purification systems, can contain excessive amounts of iron, sulfur or fluoride, can draw lead or copper from the pipes, and on occasion he contaminated with bacteria and waste products from occasional flooding.

For The Cleanse Program, I recommend using filtered or bottled water so you can have the lowest possible exposure to industrial and environmental chemicals. Of course, the final decision is always up to you.

CLEANSE FOR BEGINNERS SHOPPING LIST

The focus of your grocery shopping should be on fresh, seasonal and whole foods. Most of these foods live on the perimeter of your grocery store. At the end of this book you will find plenty of recipes to guide your grocery shopping. If you are a recipe rebel, have no fear! You can use the following list of food choices, the spice list and cooking techniques to make your own meal creations. Just stay within the rules, and you will be right on track.

So let's get to the nuts and bolts of shopping. Here are the acceptable foods for The Cleanse Program.

Protein

- Cold water fish: salmon, halibut, cod, mackerel, tuna, sardines, anchovies
- Shellfish
- Lean chicken
- Turkey and other fowl
- Lean red meats
- Lamb
- Game meat

Protein Powders

- Cleanse Detox Formula (available at www.CleanseTheBook.com)
- Rice Protein
- Hemp Protein
- Pea Protein

Fats

- Avocado
- Clarified butter
- Coconut milk or oil
- Cod liver oil
- Flaxseed oil
- Freshly ground flaxseed meal
- Macadamia nuts
- Olive oil, olives
- Raw nuts & seeds

Non-Starchy Vegetables

- Arugula
- Asparagus
- Bamboo shoots
- Bean sprouts
- Beet greens
- Bell peppers (red, yellow, green)
- Broccoli
- Brussels sprouts
- Cabbage
- Cassava
- Cauliflower
- Celery
- Chayote fruit
- Chicory
- Chives
- Collard greens
- Coriander
- Cucumber
- Dandelion greens
- Eggplant
- Endive
- Fennel
- Garlic
- Ginger root
- Green beans
- Hearts of palm
- Jicama (raw)
- Jalapeno peppers
- Kale

- Kohlrabi
- Lettuce
- Mushrooms
- Mustard greens
- Onions
- Parsley
- Radishes
- Radicchio
- Snap beans
- Snow peas
- Shallots
- Spinach
- Spaghetti squash
- Summer squash
- Swiss chard
- Tomatoes
- Turnip greens
- Watercress

High Fiber, Starchy Vegetables

- Artichokes
- Chick peas or garbanzo beans
- Leeks
- French beans
- Okra
- Pumpkin
- Squash (acorn, butternut, winter)
- Sweet potato or yam
- Turnips
- Beets
- Rutabaga
- Carrots and parsnips

Grains

- Amaranth
- Brown rice
- Wild rice
- Basmati
- Buckwheat
- Millet
- Quinoa
- Wild rice

Fruits

- Apples
- Berries (blackberries, blueberries, raspberries, strawberries)
- Grapefruit
- Lemons
- Limes
- Pear

SPICES

- Black pepper and white pepper
- Cayenne Pepper
- Cilantro
- Cinnamon
- Cloves
- Curcumin
- Dill
- Garlic
- Ginger Root
- Fennel
- Oregano
- Paprika
- Parsley
- Peppermint
- Rosemary
- Sage
- Sea Salt

SPICE WORLD

Spices, much like teas, are medicinal and can really make your life more interesting as well as help heal your body! Here is a little primer on the most common spices.

Garlic is a blood cleanser and may lower blood fats and cholesterol. It is a natural antibiotic and antimicrobial for bacteria, yeast, parasites and viral infections.

Cayenne pepper purifies the blood and tissues. It improves fluid elimination. In recent studies, capsasin (the compound that makes cayenne hot) has been found to manage type 2 diabetes. Cayenne may cause flushing and sweating.

Ginger root stimulates circulation and sweating and can ease an upset stomach. It also can relieve congestion. Ginger root contains a phytochemical known as gingerol that gives ginger its pungent smell. The benefit of gingerol is its ability to promote appropriate cell apoptosis (cell death), which is important to rejuvenation of cells.

Dandelion root acts as a diuretic and filters toxins. It is especially toning to the liver. Dandelion tea is a great daily additive.

Fennel is a sweet, aromatic, diuretic herb that relieves digestive problems, increases lactation, relaxes spasms and reduces inflammation with expectorant properties.

Paprika is a spicy seasoning ground from a variety of sweet red pepper (Capsicum annuum). Paprika pepper contains five to six times more vitamin C than an orange or lemon. It was the sweet red pepper where scientist Albert Szent-Györgyi first isolated vitamin C. Vitamin C is a potent immune system booster and beneficial in liver detoxification.

Licorice root is a mild laxative and improves immune function. It can be stimulating and can cause a rise in blood pressure. Licorice root is not safe for those on blood pressure medicine. Licorice root is great in tea form.

Parsley leaf flushes the kidneys and purifies the blood. Parsley contains a compound called polyacetylenes, which reacts strongly against carcinogens. It helps to regulate the body's production of prostaglandin controlling inflammation.

Oregano has an abundant of quercitin (an antioxidant) and farnesol (a phytochemical). Quercitin has been shown in test tube research to possess an ability to prevent the growth and proliferation of breast cancer cells. Oregano and its oil have anti-microbial and anti-viral properties and are useful in fighting infection.

Rosemary has a powerful phytochemical called carnasol, which assists the liver in its ability to detox cancer-causing substances.

Dill fruit and oil of dill possess stimulant, aromatic, anti-spasmodic and digestive properties.

Cilantro is a great herb for detoxing mercury from the body and can purify the blood.

Peppermint is commonly used to sooth the gastrointestinal tract by relaxing the muscles in the intestinal wall. When taken orally as tea or tablets, peppermint is also used for relieving respiratory conditions such as colds, coughing, acute respiratory difficulties, and for treating bacteria, fungal and viral infections.

Cloves are a spicy, warming herb that relieve pain; control nausea and vomiting; improve digestion; protect against internal parasites; and have strong antiseptic properties. Eugenol, a compound contained in clove, inhibits prostaglandin formation (inflammatory compounds) giving it an anti-inflammatory and analgesic effect.

Sage is used medicinally as a gargle for sore throats and for treatment with inflammation of the mouth and gums. Sage oil may also offer antibacterial, antifungal and antiviral effects.

Curcumin, the compound that gives turmeric its yellow color. This spice inhibits phase I detoxification while stimulating phase II.

Black pepper and white pepper were traditionally used in Chinese medicine as herbal agents. Black pepper is used for treating an upset stomach and bronchitis. White pepper is used orally for treating an upset stomach, malaria and cholera.

Sea Salt contains sodium. Sodium, in the form of sodium chloride, plays an important part in the primary processes of digestion and absorption. Salt activates salivary amylase. It also helps start digestion by breaking down food. In the parietal cells of the stomach wall, sodium chloride generates hydrochloric acid, one of the most important of all digestive secretions. If potassium, the counter balance to sodium, is in excess in relation to sodium, the body's enzyme pathway loses its ability to produce hydrochloric acid.

But what about High Blood Pressure and Salt?

According to Dr. Mark Houston, a renowned physician with the largest Hypertension clinic in the United States, only 30 percent of the people suffering from high blood pressure have a "salt sensitive" high blood pressure. The research of Dr. John H. Laragh, M.D., at the Hypertension Center of the New York-Cornell Medical Center, shows that the high blood pressure problem lies not in salt intake but rather in an overactive hormone system. When this system is overactive, there are high renin levels (Renin is a protein-digesting enzyme that acts in raising blood pressure.), body salt content is usually excessively reduced and thus salt starvation could occur if the patient is put on a low salt diet. On the other hand, a person who has low levels of renin, which occurs only in a third of hypertensive people, an excess of sodium will occur. Only patients in the last group need to lower their sodium intake.

What about sodium bloat? If you are consuming enough water for your body in relation to your sodium and potassium balance, and you are eating quality sodium with minerals (i.e., sea salt), you will not experience salt bloat.

COOKING METHODS

Many people may be eating the right foods, but with out proper cooking methods do not experience the full benefits of The Cleanse Program. Many of us were never taught how to cook, and so we can heat things in a microwave or boil water. We are going to change that on The Cleanse Program. Here are the different cooking methods you can use whether you use The Cleanse Recipes or not.

Get the Most from Your Lemons and Limes

First off, bigger is not always better—thinner skinned lemons and limes are the better choice. The lack of dimpling on the lemon or lime is usually a good indication of thinner skin.

Lemon or lime should be at room temperature.

- Roll the lemon on a hard, flat surface for 30 seconds to breakdown the fibrous membrane.
- Dropping the lemon or lime in hot water for two to three minutes will also assist in getting the most juice. Do no boil the lemons long-term, as it will degrade the enzymes and vitamin C.

- After warming the lemons and/or limes, you can then squeeze with a juicer or reamer.
- If you are juicing with your hand, squeeze the fruit into your cupped palm to catch the seeds and let the juice run off your hand. You will get three to four tablespoons of juice per lemon or lime.

VEGETABLE COOKING 101

Styles of Cooking: Blanching

Blanching is a great way to cook fresh and frozen vegetables while maintaining some freshness and crunchiness. Blanching can be used for any leafy greens, cruciferous, peas, lima beans, carrots and other vegetables.

Quick blanching also increases the color of vegetables that you may want to eat raw. Dropping cut broccoli florets in boiling water for a minute will bring the green to a bright green and make it more palatable.

Blanching is as easy as 1, 2, 3, 4 …

1. Select a pan that is deep enough for water to cover your food item.
2. Bring water to a boil
3. Add a pinch or more of sea salt or kosher salt to the water (brings out the green color in greens and assists in the blanching process).
4. Drop cut veggies into the water and let steep for one to three minutes based on the color and desired "doneness."

If you are cooking small kernel items such as peas, put the peas in a strainer and then dunk the strainer in the boiling water. This will make fishing the kernels out much easier and will also allow you to reuse the water to blanch other vegetables.

Styles of Cooking: Water Sauté

Water sauté is a great way to cook fresh vegetables and keep some freshness and crunchiness. Water sauté can be used for any leafy greens, cruciferous, peas, lima beans, carrots, and other vegetables. Water sauté also increases the color of vegetables that you may want to eat raw. Dropping cut broccoli florets in ½-inches of boiling water for a minute will bring the green to a bright green and make it more palatable.

Water sauté is as easy as 1, 2, 3, 4 …

1. Select a pan that is deep enough for you to sauté. A deep frying pan or sauté pan will work nicely.
2. Pour in water to cover the bottom by ½-inch and bring water to a boil.
3. Add a pinch or more sea salt or kosher salt to the water (brings out green color in greens and assists in the sautéing process).
4. Drop cut veggies into the water and let sauté for one to three minutes based on the color and desired "doneness."

Styles of Cooking: Boiling

Boiling is a great way to cook fresh and frozen vegetables and keep some freshness and crunchiness. Boiling can be used for any leafy greens, cruciferous, peas, lima beans, carrots, and other vegetables. Boiling is an especially wonderful cooking method for vegetables that are heavier, denser and require cooking to be edible like sweet potatoes, rutabaga, turnips, celery root and beets.

My pot boileth over 1, 2, 3, 4 …

1. Select a pan that is deep enough for water to cover your food item.
2. Bring water to a boil.
3. Add a pinch or more sea salt or kosher salt to the water.
4. Drop cut veggies into the water and let boil for one to three minutes based on the color and desired "doneness." Most root vegetables will be ready at fork doneness—the fork pushes through to the center easily.

If you are cooking small kernel items such peas, put the peas in a strainer and then dunk the strainer in the boiling water. It will make fishing the kernels out much easier and will also allow you to reuse the water to boil other vegetables.

Styles of Cooking: Roasting

Especially in the winter time, roasting is an excellent way to bring out the flavorful nuances in the foods and still cook in a healthy way. Roasting can be used for heavier more dense vegetables like sweet potatoes, red peppers, green peppers, onions, celery root and beets.

Seven simple steps to roasting …

1. Select a baking pan that is deep enough to keep the vegetables in the pan but lets them have enough room to sit in a single layer.
2. Preheat oven to 400°–450°
3. Wash and cut the vegetables into uniform chunks to aid in uniform cooking.
4. Arrange vegetables in a single layer on the bottom of the pan.
5. Drizzle with olive oil and sprinkle with sea salt and black pepper. You can always add other spices to change the flavor. I like cayenne or fresh garlic.
6. Bake for 30–40 minutes, or until the vegetables get a nice crust and browned.
7. Turn vegetables one to two times to keep the veggies from sticking to the pan.

Roasting times and temperatures may vary according to the size of the cut vegetables and oven differences.

Styles of Cooking: Grilling

Grilling is especially nice in the summer time. We like to be outside and get a little closer to our hunter/gatherer roots cooking over open fire. Grilling can be a quick method to getting food on the table. One major caveat to grilling is that an open smoking flame is going to increase the carcinogens in the food as you retain some of the fumes of the smoke in the food. So for the detox, you want to use other methods for cooking your food. However, after the detox, you may add grilling back in periodically as a cooking method.

You can reduce the toxicity of grilling considerably by cooking with wood and letting it cook down to embers rather than open flame. Gas and charcoal are less desirable because they are filled with chemicals that get deposited on your food. Keep a spray bottle nearby to douse water over open flames to keep the smoking to a minimum as well.

Vegetables are a great item to add to your grilling repertoire. The only real rules are that the vegetables need to be firm enough to hold their shape; they should also be able to lay on the grill or in a basket without falling through to the heat source. Grilling baskets are great for this purpose.

Come on Baby Light my Fire…

1. Start the fire and let it burn down to embers. The embers are very hot, so

cooking will be just as fast as an open flame. If you use an accelerant to start the fire such as lighting fluid, give the fire 15–20 minutes to burn off the residue.

2. Cut into similar sized pieces.
3. Wash and cut vegetables with the same heaviness and density into uniform chunks to aid in uniform cooking.
4. Drizzle with olive oil and sprinkle with sea salt and black pepper. You can always add other spices to change the flavor. I like cayenne or fresh garlic.
5. Arrange vegetables in a single layer on the bottom of grilling basket, or you can also skewer the vegetables into kebobs, or if they are big enough pieces, lightly spray them with olive oil and set them directly on the grate.
6. Grill until the vegetables get a nice crust and browned.
7. Turn one to two times to keep the veggies from sticking.

Grilling times and temperatures may vary according to the size of the cut vegetables and oven differences.

THE CLEANSE PROGRAM DAILY REGIMEN

The following three steps should be completed every day while on The Cleanse Program. Many people choose to continue with this regimen post-cleanse.

Step 1: Hydration and Lymphatic Stimulant

Daily Hydration: Flushing your system and reducing sugar cravings

- Mix 2-ounces of organic, un-sweetened cranberry, un-sweetened pomegranate, black cherry or un-sweetened acai juice with 32-ounces of water equaling a MINIMUM of 34-ounces. Drink this beverage throughout the day. The beverage should be pink, not deep red in color.
- Drink an additional 64-ounces of filtered or spring water at room temperature or warm with lemon and lime juice if you would like a little flavor.
- You may drink two to four cups of herbal teas to aid in detoxification. These can count toward your regular water intake as long as they do not contain caffeine. I enjoy red clover and licorice tea.

Step 2: Gut Healing Morning Smoothie/Pudding

- Take ½-cup of organic applesauce with or without cinnamon.
- Add one to three tablespoons ground flax meal or PaleoFiber.
- Add one tablespoon glutamine powder for extra healing. This is especially beneficial for the Advance recipes users.
- Mix all ingredients together and then enjoy as a pudding or use the mixed ingredients as a base for a morning smoothie with protein powder added.

Step 3: Putting Out the Inflammation Fire

Take one tablespoon of flax oil either in your Gut Healing Smoothie, or use it to make salad dressings. You can also just take a tablespoon a day.

THE CLEANSE PROGRAM FOODS

Non-Vegetarians

- VEGETABLES! Increase vegetables, especially leafy greens. Eat at least five to seven servings a day (1-cup raw or ½-cup cooked).
- Eat lean proteins (fish, fowl, buffalo, game and lean red meat).
- Eat vegetable soups for lunch or dinner to rest digestion. you can find several recipes in the advanced recipe section (great for lunch).
- Supplement protein intake with Cleanse Detox Formula or rice protein shakes made with berries.
- Increase omega-3 fat intake by adding flax oil daily on steamed vegetables.
- Eat tree nuts (walnuts, almonds and pecans) as long as you are not allergic to increase good fats.
- Eat an apple a day for additional fiber.
- You may need to eat five to six small meals throughout the day. If you have blood sugar management issues, you will probably get hungry more frequently. If you do not have blood sugar issues, you may find three to four meals are perfect for you.
- You may have one servings (½-cup) of brown rice, millet, quinoa or amaranth grain in its natural cooked form each day. Try and limit the grain intake and use vegetables instead.
- Root vegetables such as beets, carrots, turnips and rutabaga are all great choices

for vegetable forms of starch.
- Drink green, white or black tea to wean yourself off coffee and other stimulants.
- Drink two to four herbal teas a day to improve the detoxification process.
- Use stevia or xylitol to sweeten foods. Moderation is key.

Vegetarians

- VEGETABLES! Increase vegetables, especially leafy greens. Eat at least five to seven servings a day (1-cup raw or ½-cup cooked).
- Supplement protein with Cleanse Detox Formula or Hemp protein powder. Do not use soy, whey or casein powders.
- Eat vegetable soups to rest digestion (great for lunch).
- Supplement protein intake with rice protein shakes made with berries.
- Increase omega-3 fat intake by adding flax oil daily on steamed vegetables.
- Eat tree nuts (walnuts, almonds and pecans) as long as you are not allergic to increase good fats.
- Eat an apple a day for additional fiber.
- You may need to eat five to six small meals throughout the day. If you have blood sugar management issues, you will probably get hungry more frequently. If you do not have blood sugar issues, you may find three to four meals are perfect for you.
- You may have one to two servings (½-cup) of brown rice, millet, quinoa or amaranth grain in its natural cooked form a day. Try and limit the grain intake and use vegetables instead.
- Root vegetables such as beets, carrots, turnips and rutabaga are all great choices for vegetable forms of starch.
- Eat one to two ½-cup servings of black beans, garbanzo beans, lentils, black-eyed peas, azuki/aduki beans, field peas and green peas for protein.
- Drink green, white or black tea to wean yourself off coffee and other stimulants.
- Drink one to four cups herbal teas each day to improve the detoxification process.
- Use stevia, or xylitol to sweeten foods.

FOODS NOT ALLOWED ON THE CLEANSE PROGRAM

You will be removing all of the top allergen foods: soy, wheat and gluten-containing grains, dairy, sugar, citrus (except lemon, lime and grapefruit) and high sugar fruits, yeast, peanuts, eggs and corn.

- No dairy foods: milk, cheese, yogurt, ice cream and cream, half and half.
- No high-glycemic sugar fruits: pineapple, banana, melons and mangos.
- No wheat or gluten-containing grains: wheat, cereal, wheat berries, spelt, bulgur, rye, tricale, pasta and breads.
- No peanuts: Peanuts are not actually nuts.
- No soy foods: tofu, tempeh and soy sauce.
- No orange or tangerine citrus.
- No oatmeal; it is usually processed in plants where wheat is processed.
- No eggs or foods containing eggs.
- No sugar: sugar cane, beet sugar, sucanat, turbinado, powdered sugar.
- No coffee, diet drinks or sodas of any kind.
- No chips, crackers, pasta, cereals, breads, tortillas or processed foods.
- No artificial chemical flavors, sweeteners or additives.

Remove Sugar, Alcohol, Caffeine and Toxic Chemicals

All of the above mentioned "food stuff"—I hesitate to call it food—are hard on the body as you well know by now! So as a quickie reminder: Sugar depletes the body of minerals. In order to be broken down, the body will leech minerals from bones and tissues. Alcohol must be cleansed by the liver and causes substantial damage to the liver tissue. It preferentially gets absorbed and converted to sugar over food and goes straight to the belly in the form of fat. Fake sweeteners such as Aspartame, Saccharin and Sucralose are neurotoxins that damage the nervous system and lead to mood, cognitive and behavioral disorders. Caffeine is a psychoactive drug that can cause damage to the central nervous system, and leads to addiction and adrenal stress. Yes, coffee beans do have some good values but we are going to take it out for the purpose of The Cleanse Program.

Remove Gluten-Containing Grains

Gluten-containing grains have an amino acid complex called gliadin that is indigestible by man. In a substantial part of the population, gliadin causes an immune response that will damage the small intestines causing intestinal permeability, malnourishment and a host of other disorders. Gliadin has a peptide component called gluto-morphine that crosses the blood-brain barrier exerting neurological damage and mood disorders. For some people it is not the "staff of life"

Remove all forms of Dairy

Many people are sensitive to the casein found in dairy (cheese), as well as whey protein. Casein sensitivities play a heavy role in mood and cognitive disorders, digestive and allergy disorders. Dairy causes excess mucus and exacerbates allergies and skin breakouts. Remember our discussion of dairy from earlier in the book? I promise many of you will thank me after your cleanse is over. Dairy is often a culprit in long-lasting problems with digestion, allergies, skin and breathing disorders.

Remove Highly Acidic Beans

Many raw beans contain a harmful toxin (Phytohaemagglutinin) that must be removed, usually by soaking and cooking in order to make the beans edible. Beans also contain high level of lectins which can activate the immune system resulting in leaky gut syndrome and food sensitivities. All edible beans contain oligosaccharides. An anti-oligosaccharide enzyme is necessary to properly digest these sugar molecules. A normal human digestive tract does not contain any anti-oligosaccharide enzymes.

For this reason, a good balance of intestinal bacteria is needed to digest beans since humans do not make an olgiosacchride digestive enzyme. People with gas and bloating after eating beans often have an out of balance ecosystem of gut bacteria resulting in the improper fermentation of the sugars in beans in the large intestines by the bacteria.

The most acidic beans are kidney, cannelli, pinto and navy beans. The Cleanse Program includes balancing the acid/alkaline balance of the diet. We will be removing these three beans from the diet.

Remove Soy Foods

Soy is one of the top five food allergens. Almost all packaged foods contain soy isolates. Soy contains a natural chemical that mimics estrogen, the female hormone. Some studies in animals show that this chemical can alter sexual development. Humans cannot digest soybeans without significant preparation such as soaking and fermentation. Only after fermentation for some time, or extensive processing, are the beans suitable for digestion.

Remove All Forms of Yeast, Fermented Foods and Fungus

Yeast in the diet increases the yeast overload often found in an out of balance gut. Yeast overgrowth may play a significant role in many disease states and symptoms. Yeast in the gut can cause sugar cravings, digestive issues and mood changes. Yeast foods can often be the cause of digestive complaints, specifically brewer's and baker's yeast. Almost all packaged foods contain yeast or yeast derivatives.

Remove all vinegars except distilled, Ume plum and apple cider vinegar.

Remove Corn

Almost all packaged foods contain corn or a corn derivative. Corn may play a role in the development of asthma, chronic bronchitis and sinus infections. Corn, like much of the above list, is often part of everything we eat it is so ubiquitous in processed foods especially when you take into account the number of foods that contain corn syrup and high fructose corn syrup or corn starch.

Many of the symptoms of a corn sensitivity mimic the symptoms of sensitivity to other foods such as digestive complaints, migraine headaches, asthma attacks and/or shortness-of-breath.

Remove Citrus: Oranges, Pineapple and High Sugar Fruits

Citrus and tropical fruits are some of the top food allergens. Citrus fruit can cause digestive distress and other digestive complaints due to the high fructose content. Many have trouble digesting the pulp, which can lead to rather unpleasant diarrhea. Citrus foods can exacerbate acid reflux, ulcers or other sourness sensitivities. Citrus foods cause problems for people with Crohn's, IBD and IBS. Citric fruits can also been found to be a culprit in rashes on the skin around the lips or sores inside the mouth. Additionally, citrus juices are high in sugar and can wreak havoc on your blood sugar control!

Remove Anything Processed

Processing—making a whole food into a processed food—destroys nutrients in the foods. The milling, refining and stripping techniques refine all nutritive portions such as the bran coating and seed parts leaving only the caloric carbohydrate portion behind. Oftentimes the processed food is so depleted of nutrients that the food must then be fortified so it will not cause nutrient deficiencies.

Breads, crackers, cereals, chips and pasta, cakes, cookies and man-made foods are all processed. Here is a good way to think of it: if it comes in a box or bag with a label you will not be eating it on The Cleanse Program.

3-DAY COUNTDOWN

Now that you know what to buy, let's get a timeline together! Planning is where most people derail on the path to health and wellness. So do not skip this step, as it is vital to your success.

Go through the recipes in the back of the book to determine what meals you want make. You do not have to use the recipes included, but they have been crafted to remove all of the items not on The Cleanse Program without sacrificing the taste.

I always start the cleanse on a Sunday, which gives me a chance to use the weekend as prep days one and two. This schedule also allows me to get the first day under my belt before the workweek starts. Choose when you want to start based on your own lifestyle and schedule.

Prep Day 1

Reduce coffee consumption. You may go half caffeine-free or substitute green tea for coffee. This is also the day to make a conscious step towards reducing sugar consumption.

Shop for the following items:

- Unsweetened pomegranate or acai juice
- Stevia or xylitol sweeteners
- Filtered or bottled water
- Lemons and limes
- Spices and fresh herbs

- Variety of vegetables
- A variety of green leafy vegetables
- Tubers: sweet potatoes, beets, yams, carrots, etc.
- Cruciferous vegetables: broccoli, cabbage, cauliflower
- Flavoring vegetables: Onions, garlic, celery, cilantro, parsley
- Coconut Oil for cooking
- Flax oil (in the refrigerated section of most health food stores)
- Olive oil, avocado or walnut oil
- Organic fish, chicken and turkey
- Brown rice, quinoa and millet grain
- Almond or cashew butter
- Unsweetened almond milk, (unless allergic to almonds), coconut, rice milk, hazelnut or hemp milk (found in the milk section of the grocery store). Choose from the following brands: So Delicous, Almond breeze, Pacific and Hemp Bliss, respectively.

Quality nutritional supplements are not easy to find. Most of the industry is unregulated, and therefore, supplements can be filled with less than quality fillers and chemicals. I have sourced what I believe to be the best rice protein powder supplemental food, which is the most hypo-allergenic of all sources. You are not required to use The Cleanse Detox Formula; however, it will save you time and effort in finding quality choices. Purchase Cleanse Detox Formula at www.CleanseTheBook.com.

THE CLEANSE PROGRAM FOOD

If you choose to shop on your own, you want to select a rice, pea, hemp or as a last resort, a whey protein powder. For the fiber, you may buy flax meal or flax seed as a fiber source. If you buy the seed, you will need to grind it in a coffee grinder to make the seed usable.

Prep Day 2

- Day two should be a big preparation day. Please take this time to get your kitchen, and your life, in order.
- Make a few jugs of unsweetened cranberry, pomegranate juice or acai and

water combination.

- Ground a portion of the flax seed and store in an air-tight container in the refrigerator.
- Clean vegetables for your meals throughout the week.
- Clean and chop green leafy vegetables.
- Clean and prep tubers: sweet potatoes, beets, yams, and carrots for easy preparation.
- Clean and chop cruciferous vegetables: broccoli, cabbage, cauliflower.
- Wash and store flavoring vegetables: onions, garlic, celery, cilantro, parsley (cilantro and parsley store well standing in a glass of water with the plastic bag draped over the top).
- Pre-bake, steam, saute, or grill several protein choices for lunches and dinner.
- Cook several servings of grains for fast reheating.
- Prepare a soup recipe for quick snacks or meals.

You are now ready to go.

SAMPLE DAY ON THE CLEANSE PROGRAM

You do not have to follow this menu guideline exactly but you can use the general gist of it to tailor the menus to your desires. The important thing to watch is the combinations of foods and the removal of foods during the progression of the Cleanse. Just a word to the wise, if you are not a big water drinker, I find spreading the water and juice mixture out throughout the day is better than trying to chug it all late at night. Heed that warning: you may spend a lot more time in the bathroom at night if you do not.

CLEANSE WEEK ONE

This week you will concentrate on adding in good things: hydrating drink: water with cranberry juice combination and extra water today. I recommend having 20 ounces of the cranberry water mixture upon waking and have a big glass before each meal.

And removing the foods, additives and chemicals in your diet: remove coffee, sodas and diet drinks, all forms of added sugar, fake sweeteners, cow dairy and gluten containing grains, eggs, yeast, citrus, high-sugar fruits, soy, peanuts and acidic beans.

Day One

Breakfast

- 1 serving of Gut Healing Pudding with 1 tbsp Flax and 2 tbsp L-Glutamine
- ¾ Morning No Oat Meal
- 2 ounce Chicken Breakfast sausage
- 1 cup green Tea

Lunch

- 2 cups tossed green salad with 4 oz. grilled chicken and 2 tablespoon Tahini dressing
- Snack
- ¼ cup of hummus with cut red pepper as a dipping "chips"
- 1 cup Red clover tea

Dinner

- 1 cup Thai Pumpkin Soup
- 6-ounces of Broiled Sole with Lemon
- 2 cups Spinach Caesar salad
- Bedtime
- 1 cup of chamomile tea

Day Two

Breakfast

- 1 serving of Gut Healing Pudding with 1 tbsp Flax and 2 tbsp L-Glutamine
- ¾ Quinoa Porridge
- 2 ounce Chicken Breakfast sausage
- 1 cup green tea

Lunch

- 2 cups Kitchen Sink Salad with 2 tablespoons olive oil and lime dressing
- 6 ounces (leftover) Baked Sole with Lemon

Snack

- ¼ cup of hummus with cut red pepper as a dipping "chips"
- 1 cup green tea

Dinner

- 6-ounces Chicken Mole
- ½ cup Amaranth grits
- 1 cup simmered Greens with Onions

Bedtime

- 1 cup of chamomile tea

Day Three

Breakfast

- 1 serving of Gut Healing Pudding with 1 tbsp Flax and 2 tbsp L-Glutamine
- ¾ Quinoa Porridge
- 2 ounce Chicken Breakfast sausage
- 1 cup green tea

Lunch

- 2 cups Thai Pumpkin Soup
- 2 cup green salad with Tahini Dressing

Snack

- ¼ cup of hummus with cut red pepper as a dipping "chips"
- 1 cup green tea

Dinner

- 6-ounces Herb Marinated Chicken
- ½ cup Amaranth grits
- 1 cup Stir Fried vegetables

Bedtime

- 1 cup of chamomile tea

Day Four

Breakfast

- 1 serving of Gut Healing Pudding with 1 tbsp Flax and 2 tbsp L-Glutamine
- ¾ cup Quinoa Porridge
- 2 ounce Chicken Breakfast sausage
- 1 cup green Tea

Lunch

- 2 cups Curry-tastic Soup
- 1 large apple with 2 tablespoons almond butter
- Snack
- ¼ cup of hummus with cut red pepper as a dipping "chips"
- 1 cup Red clover tea

Dinner

- 6-ounces of Herb Marinated Chicken (breast)
- Cinnamon Baked Squash
- 2 cups Broccoli Rabe with Caramelized Onions and Garlic

Bedtime

- 1 cup of chamomile tea

Day Five

Breakfast

- 1 serving of Gut Healing Pudding with 1 tbsp Flax and 2 tbsp L-Glutamine
- 1 cup Cinnamon Baked Squash
- 1 cup green tea

Lunch

- 2 cups Cari-Bean Salad
- 1 large apple with 2 tablespoons almond butter

Snack

- ½ salsa with cut vegetables

- 1 cup green tea

Dinner

- 6-ounces Chicken Walnut Stir-Fry
- ½ cup brown rice
- 1 cup sautéed leeks and cabbage

Bedtime

- 1 cup of chamomile tea

Day Six

Breakfast

- 1 serving of Gut Healing Pudding with 1 tbsp Flax and 2 tbsp L-Glutamine
- Power Millet (use leftover brown rice) Shake
- 1 cup green tea

Lunch

- 2 cups Kitchadi soup
- 1 cup Collards with Dill and Parsley

Snack

- ¼ cup of hummus with cut red pepper as a dipping "chips"
- 1 cup green tea

Dinner

- 6-ounces Herb Marinated Chicken Breast
- Roasted Root Vegetables
- 1 cup simmered Greens with Onions

Bedtime

- 1 cup of chamomile tea

Day Seven

Breakfast

- 1 serving of Gut Healing Pudding with 1 tbsp Flax and 2 tbsp L-Glutamine

- ¾ cup Quinoa Porridge
- 1 cup green tea

Lunch

- 2 cups Thai Pumpkin Soup
- 1 large apple with 2 tablespoons almond butter

Snack

- ¼ cup walnuts
- 1 cup green tea

Dinner

- 6-ounces baked chicken breast
- Zesty Quinoa with Broccoli and Cashews

Bedtime

- 1 cup of chamomile tea

CLEANSE WEEK TWO

Now that we have a much cleaner diet and better functioning digestive system, we can ramp up our detoxification process by including two servings daily of our Cleanse Detox Formula food shakes. We are also going to be cutting back on the grain servings while increasing vegetables.

Day Eight

Breakfast

- 1 serving of Gut Healing Pudding with 1 tbsp Flax and 2 tbsp L-Glutamine
- Basic Fruit Shake with The Cleanse Detox Formula and ½ cup Strawberries
- 1 cup green Tea

Snack

- 1 large apple with 2 tablespoons almond butter
- 1 cup Red clover tea

Lunch

- 2 cups Ginger Sweet Potato Soup with Cilantro

- 1 cup steamed spinach with 2 tablespoon Tahini dressing

Snack

- ¼ cup of hummus with cut red pepper as a dipping "chips"
- 1 cup Red clover tea

Dinner

- 6-ounces of Broiled Sole with Lemon
- ½ cup Italian Style Garbanzo Beans
- 2 cups Spinach Caesar salad

Bedtime

- The Cleanse Detox Formula in 1 cup almond milk and 2 tbsp almond butter
- 1 cup of chamomile tea

Day Nine

Breakfast

- 1 serving of Gut Healing Pudding with 1 tbsp Flax and 2 tbsp L-Glutamine
- Basic Fruit Shake with The Cleanse Detox Formula in 1 cup almond milk and ½ cup frozen Strawberries
- 1 cup green tea

Lunch

- 2 cups Kitchen Sink Salad with 2 tablespoons olive oil and lime dressing
- 6 ounces (leftover) Baked Chicken Breast

Snack

- ¼ cup of hummus with cut red pepper as a dipping "chips"
- 1 cup green tea

Dinner

- 6-ounces Chipotle Chicken and Butternut Squash Soup
- 2 cup Green Salad with Tahini Dressing

Bedtime

- The Cleanse Detox Formula in 1 cup almond milk and 2 tbsp almond butter
- 1 cup of chamomile tea

Day Ten

Breakfast

- 1 serving of Gut Healing Pudding with 1 tbsp Flax and 2 tbsp L-Glutamine
- Basic Almond Butter Shake
- 1 cup green tea

Lunch

- 2 cups Creamy Broccoli Soup
- 6 ounces Baked Chicken

Snack

- ¼ cup of hummus with cut red pepper as a dipping "chips"
- 1 cup green tea

Dinner

- 6-ounces Orange Roughy and Scallions with Ginger
- 2 cup Stir Fry Vegetables

Bedtime

- The Cleanse Detox Formula in 1 cup almond milk and 2 tbsp almond butter
- 1 cup of chamomile tea

Day Eleven

Breakfast

- 1 serving of Gut Healing Pudding with 1 tbsp Flax and 2 tbsp L-Glutamine
- Breakfast Berry Compote
- 1 cup green Tea

Snack

- 1 large apple with 2 tablespoons almond butter
- 1 cup Red clover tea

Lunch

- 2 cups Aduki Bean Soup
- 1 large apple with 2 tablespoons almond butter

Snack

- ¼ cup of hummus with cut red pepper as a dipping "chips"
- 1 cup Red clover tea

Dinner

- 6-ounces of Herb Marinated Chicken (breast)
- Spicy Kale-Almond Pesto and Chickpea Ratatouli

Bedtime

- Basic Fruit Shake with The Cleanse Detox Formula and ½ cup Strawberries
- 1 cup of chamomile tea

Day Twelve

Breakfast

- 1 serving of Gut Healing Pudding with 1 tbsp Flax and 2 tbsp L-Glutamine
- Basic Fruit Shake with Peaches
- 1 cup green tea

Lunch

- 2 cups Lucky Lucy Salad
- 1 large apple with 2 tablespoons almond butter

Snack

- ½ salsa with cut vegetables
- 1 cup green tea

Dinner

- 6-ounces Roasted Salmon and Stir Fry Vegetables
- 1 cup Hot Spot Greens

Bedtime

- The Cleanse Detox Formula in 1 cup almond milk and 2 tbsp almond butter
- 1 cup of chamomile tea

Day Thirteen

Breakfast

- 1 serving of Gut Healing Pudding with 1 tbsp Flax and 2 tbsp L-Glutamine
- Basic Fruit Shake with Strawberries
- 1 cup green tea

Snack

- 1 large apple with 2 tablespoons almond butter
- 1 cup Red clover tea

Lunch

- 2 cups Summer Salad with Avocado Salad Dressing
- 6 ounce broiled Sole with Lemon

Snack

- ¼ cup of hummus with cut red pepper as a dipping "chips"
- 1 cup green tea

Dinner

- 6-ounces baked chicken breast
- Roasted Root Vegetables
- 2 cup kale Potato chips

Bedtime

- The Cleanse Detox Formula in 1 cup almond milk and 2 tbsp almond butter
- 1 cup of chamomile tea

Day Fourteen

Breakfast

- 1 serving of Gut Healing Pudding with 1 tbsp Flax and 2 tbsp L-Glutamine
- Basic Fruit Shake with ½ cup Blueberries
- 1 cup green tea

Lunch

- 2 cups Salsa Salad

- 1 large apple with 2 tablespoons almond butter

Snack

- ¼ cup walnuts
- 1 cup green tea

Dinner

- 6-ounces Chicken Piccata
- Sautéed Spinach with Caramelized Onions

Bedtime

- The Cleanse Detox Formula in 1 cup almond milk
- 1 cup of chamomile tea

CLEANSE WEEK THREE

This week we will slowly work our way to a less stringent eating plan reintroducing non-gluten containing grains back into the diet and reducing the cleansing Cleanse Detox Formula food to one serving a day. At the end of week three, you will slowly begin to add back the toxic 8 foods one at a time that we removed to determine if any of those foods are causing symptoms.

Day Fifteen

Breakfast

- 1 serving of Gut Healing Pudding with 1 tbsp Flax and 2 tbsp L-Glutamine
- Basic Fruit Shake with The Cleanse Detox Formula and ½ cup Strawberries
- 1 cup green Tea

Snack

- 1 large apple with 2 tablespoons almond butter
- 1 cup Red clover tea

Lunch

- 2 cups Ginger Sweet Potato Soup with Cilantro
- 1 cup steamed spinach with 2 tablespoon Tahini dressing

Snack

- ¼ cup of hummus with cut red pepper as a dipping "chips"
- 1 cup Red clover tea

Dinner

- 6-ounces of Broiled Sole with Lemon
- ½ cup Italian Style Garbanzo Beans
- 2 cups Spinach Caesar salad

Bedtime

- 1 cup of chamomile tea

Day Sixteen

Breakfast

- 1 serving of Gut Healing Pudding with 1 tbsp Flax and 2 tbsp L-Glutamine
- Basic Fruit Shake with The Cleanse Detox Formula and ½ cup Strawberries
- 1 cup green tea

Lunch

- 2 cups Kitchen Sink Salad with 2 tablespoons olive oil and lime dressing
- 6 ounces (leftover) Baked Chicken Breast

Snack

- ¼ cup of hummus with cut red pepper as a dipping "chips"
- 1 cup green tea

Dinner

- 6-ounces Chicken Piccata
- 1 cup Spinach Caesar Salad
- 1 cup Italian-Style Garbanzo Beans

Bedtime

- 1 cup of chamomile tea

Day Seventeen

Breakfast

- 1 serving of Gut Healing Pudding with 1 tbsp Flax and 2 tbsp L-Glutamine
- Basic Almond Butter Shake
- 1 cup green tea

Lunch

- 2 cups Kitchen Sink salad with Basic Italian Dressing
- 6 ounces Baked Chicken

Snack

- ¼ cup of hummus with cut red pepper as a dipping "chips"
- 1 cup green tea

Dinner

- 6-ounces Orange Roughy and Scallions with Ginger
- 2 cup Stir Fry Vegetables
- ½ cup brown rice

Bedtime

- Basic Fruit Shake with Blueberries
- 1 cup of chamomile tea

Day Eighteen

Breakfast

- 1 serving of Gut Healing Pudding with 1 tbsp Flax and 2 tbsp L-Glutamine
- Breakfast Berry Compote
- 1 cup green Tea

Snack

- 1 large apple with 2 tablespoons almond butter
- 1 cup Red clover tea

Lunch

- 2 Baked Stuffed Green Peppers

- 1 large apple with 2 tablespoons almond butter

Snack

- ¼ cup of hummus with cut red pepper as a dipping "chips"
- 1 cup Red clover tea

Dinner

- 6-ounces of Herb Marinated Chicken (breast)
- 1 cup steamed broccoli
- ½ cup Amaranth grits

Bedtime

- 1 cup of chamomile tea

Day Nineteen

Breakfast

- 1 serving of Gut Healing Pudding with 1 tbsp Flax and 2 tbsp L-Glutamine
- Basic Fruit Shake with Peaches
- 1 cup green tea

Lunch

- Spicy Kale-Almond Pesto and Chickpea Ratatouille
- ½ brown rice

Snack

- ½ salsa with cut vegetables
- 1 cup green tea

Dinner

- 6-ounces Chicken and Rice
- 1 cup Sautéed Green Beans

Bedtime

- Basic Fruit Shake with Peaches
- 1 cup of chamomile tea

Day Twenty

Breakfast

- 1 serving of Gut Healing Pudding with 1 tbsp Flax and 2 tbsp L-Glutamine
- Basic Fruit Shake with Strawberries
- 1 cup green tea

Snack

- 1 large apple with 2 tablespoons almond butter
- 1 cup Red clover tea

Lunch

- 2 cups Crunchy Quinoa Salad
- 6 ounce broiled Sole with Lemon
- Snack
- ¼ cup of hummus with cut red pepper as a dipping "chips"
- 1 cup green tea

Dinner

- 6-ounces baked chicken breast
- 1 cup Steamed Green Beans
- 1 cup boiled red Potatoes

Bedtime

- 1 cup of chamomile tea

Day Twenty-One

Breakfast

- 1 serving of Gut Healing Pudding with 1 tbsp Flax and 2 tbsp L-Glutamine
- Sweet Potato Pancakes
- 1 cup green tea

Lunch

- 2 cups Salsa Salad
- 1 large apple with 2 tablespoons almond butter

Snack

- 1 large pear and ¼ cup walnuts
- 1 cup green tea

Dinner

- 6-ounces Chicken Piccata
- ½ cup Amaranth grits
- Broccoli Rabe with Caramelized Onions and Garlic

Bedtime

- 1 cup of chamomile tea

EXTRA MEASURES TO INCREASE CLEANSING

- Use the recipes for blended soups and blended vegetable shakes to replace at least one meal a day or use as a snack.
- Increase fiber intake by sprinkling flax meal on steamed vegetables.
- Add fish oil, a digestive enzymes and herbal teas to improve digestion.
- Add a serving of powdered greens to your water with lime for extra antioxidants.
- Add regular, sweaty exercise (walk, yoga) or saunas to your daily regimen to improve toxin removal.

ADVANCED RECIPES FOR CLEANSING

Some people may either be ready for cleansing at a deeper level, or perhaps are maybe the classic over-achiever who wants to go all the way. So, if you want to kick The Cleanse Program up a notch, here are the things to focus on to ramp up the detoxification:

- Use the advanced recipes for blended soups and blended vegetable shakes to replace at least one meal a day or use as a snack.
- Replace two meals, or a meal and a snack, with Cleanse Detox Formula shake using the shake recipes in the back.
- Make your evening meal the only solid food you eat and have that meal contain two non-starchy vegetable sides, or a big salad with one starchy vegetable and a 6-ounce portion of protein.
- Increase fiber intake by sprinkling flax meal on salad and steamed vegetables

Add fish oil, digestive enzymes and herbal teas to improve digestion

- Add a serving of powdered greens to your water with lime for extra antioxidants.
- Add regular sweaty exercise (walk, yoga, etc.) or saunas to your daily regimen to improve toxin removal.

    Now that you have made it through the "whys" and "hows," you are ready to rock and roll. Okay, enough reading—get started! We will meet back in chapter 12 for the exciting process of coming off The Cleanse Program.

12
Coming Off Cleanse

> *Health is a state of complete physical, mental and social well-being, and not merely the absence of disease or infirmity.*
> *- World Health Organization, 1948*

JEFF GORA, TESTIMONIAL

When I started The Cleanse Program workshop, I just knew that I was setting my body up for some positive changes. Not only had I seen my wife realize the benefits while participating in The Cleanse Program, I also knew that I had never taken my nutrition, and subsequently my general eating habits, very seriously. Within the first two hours of the "kickoff" class, I gained a substantial amount of knowledge regarding how my body reacted to the foods I ate. Armed with this new awareness and the assurance that the benefit would be quickly realized, I felt confident to start the process.

Initially, I was concerned that I would not be able to muster the discipline necessary to change my diet, but I quickly realized that the program is designed to bring the body, as quickly as possible, into a state of nutritional balance that naturally staves off the cravings and temptations that I have experienced when dieting only for weight loss. The combination of eating the right foods (as outlined through the program) and timing my meals per the plan, fueled my body to a point of high efficiency.

My increased energy was remarkable. I slept better, felt mentally sharper, was more comfortable during exercise and even seemed to suffer less from some of common ailments such as hay fever and allergies.

I also noticed that by following the recommended food list and timing my meals as designed, I took in much fewer calories each day than I had previously, though my body felt to be fueled so much better. I never felt hungry. Through all the excitement of this general improvement in my health, it was not lost on me that I was beginning to see a comfortable loss of weight as well. I was very excited to realize that over the three-week period I had lost seventeen pounds, an added benefit to having cleansed and fueled my system to a point of such high efficiency.

I was so encouraged by my results that I decided to stay with the plan for a total of eight weeks. The extension was somewhat effortless for me, being buoyed by such a noticeable improvement in my health. I was eating healthy, real foods that made me feel great.

Having reintroducing many of the foods I had eliminated back into my diet, I now have a very good feel for what items have what effect on my general health. I am also proud to say that I am enjoying the positive side effect of a 40 pound weight loss over the eight weeks and a much more positive outlook on my life.

CATHY BROOKS-FINE, TESTIMONIAL

The Cleanse Program was a launch pad for a new, healthier way of eating. Removing chemicals, additives and other harmful substances that inhibit my well-being was a New Year's Resolution and this program worked into my plan perfectly. It was great to eliminate the toxic clutter of everyday living.

While on the program I did notice some side effects of food and toxins on my system and also became more aware of my thirst threshold. I was constantly thirsty even though I was drinking much more water than normal. I realized that I had been depriving my body of water. I experienced some minor acne issues as toxins were released. I decided to follow the advice about sweating and took a trip to a local Russian Banya (Bath House), which expedited my detoxification process.

I lost three pounds during The Cleanse Program and had a 4 percent decrease in my body fat, but the most dramatic change was in how I felt. I felt lighter, had more energy and was able to exercise longer with less muscle fatigue. I felt as though I had given my body a clean slate.

Unfortunately, I found that I did have reactions to some of my favorite foods. I love cheese, but I now know that dairy is not my friend. I am more cognizant about when and how much I consume it. I also know the consequences should I indulge.

After experiencing The Cleanse Program, in general, I am a healthier eater. I feel empowered by the knowledge I gained on this program, and I am now able to truly listen to my body and do what is best for it. I seriously consider what I put into my now clean body. Also, the recipes provided with the program are easy to follow and have been incorporated into my family's daily meal repertoire.

DAY 22 AND BEYOND

As you know, there is nothing magic about the 21 days of cleansing. Why stop now? You may choose to stay on The Cleanse Program for a longer period of time to improve health outcomes, improve weight loss and continue feeling a reduction in negative symptoms. You could even stay on The Cleanse Program long-term. Many of my Cleansers have stayed on it for six or more months at a time. You have not removed any food groups. You have optimized nutrition by eating whole, organic foods and reduced your exposure to toxins and toxic chemicals.

Is there any harm in coming out of the Cleanse incorrectly? The real answer is yes and no. I have had people just jump off the deep end and binge on day 22 of The Cleanse Program. Some of these "deep-enders" experienced a significant reaction. Most had digestive upset while their body tried to handle the toxic load of pizza and beer. So, yes you may potentially have digestive upset or other hangover type of symptoms.

The most important component of coming off The Cleanse Program is to not undo all of the good work that resulted in positive changes. You want to maintain the ability to determine which foods cause you discomfort. You may not be "sensitive" to any of the removed foods; however, you may find that these foods in larger doses are not giving you the health and body that you desire.

The Cleanse Program is about discernment and learning long-term, realistic changes that you can make to improve your health and wellbeing. You have cleaned up your diet in a way that can really work for you. Continuing to eat a diet of whole foods will be beneficial to help you on your way to a lifetime of optimal health.

Cleansing for weight loss tends to foster an exploration of many other aspects about the individual, not just the physical. Rather than focusing on a a "weight issue," Cleansers begin to examine the emotional suppression that is underlying the excess pounds. They begin to unfold more and connect with hidden parts of themselves, reaching out to others for support. Far from being a process of losing some fat and water then reverting to old habits, this cleanse is about positive, real life changes. Working through these shifts may feel tough in the short-term, but over time will leave you clearer and less likely to return to self-destructive patterns.

EATING THE "CLEANSE WAY" CONTINUALLY

Whole foods are edible substances as close to their "whole" or natural state as possible. They have not been pre-processed in any way that would disturb their nutritional value, nutrient content or flavor. Whole foods are, therefore, free of all processing additives or subtractions. The Cleanse is a whole foods eating plan. The overall idea of whole foods, is to buy foods that meet the following criteria:

- Foods that are in their most simple and natural form.
- Foods that are in season and from as close to the source as possible.
- Foods that are as chemical and additive free as possible.
- Foods that are sold in bulk and not pre-packaged.
- Foods that are free from pesticides, herbicides and hormones.

LIFE BEYOND CLEANSING

For many people, the end of The Cleanse Program is bittersweet. They feel better than they ever have in their adult life. Many nagging symptoms of a clogged, overloaded digestion and detoxification system have resolved into a cleaner, leaner running body. And yet, some may people still have emotional attachments to unhealthy foods and may be dreaming of their next pizza and beer or a glass of wine and sugary dessert. Please, before you go off the deep end and dive right back in the junk food pool, read on to learn a few more things about your body!

When you are ready to return to "regular" eating, begin to slowly add foods back into the diet. Since you have eliminated several foods that may be causing reactions in your body, you need slowly reintroduce each food so you can discern any responses you may be having from each particular food.

RULES OF FOOD REINTRODUCTION

The reintroduction plan reintroduces foods in the order in which previous Cleanser indicated they most wanted. You can rearrange the food groups in whatever way you desire. Just do not to mix food categories. If you experience symptoms, do not introduce another food category until your symptom has subsided.

INTRODUCTION OF DAIRY: DAY 22-24

Select one dairy item to add back. Cheese would be ideal to start with since it is comprised of casein, the component of dairy most associated with symptoms. If you are not a fan of cheese, you may want to choose milk. If you do not eat dairy, then proceed to the next food group. Start by introducing a serving of dairy back into your day as a snack alone or as a component of a meal. Over the next three days, you can add two to three servings of dairy each day.

Keep a Reintroducing Foods Journal and answer the following questions each time you eat a food you are reintroducing to your diet.

- Does your body feel different now?
- How does your body feel three hours after eating the reintroduced food?
- How does your body feel one day after eating the reintroduced food?
- How does your body feel three days after eating the reintroduced food?
- Are you bloated, gassy, tired or foggy-headed? Are you experiencing any digestive symptoms?
- Do you have gas or are you bloating?
- Do you have diarrhea?
- Do you have constipation?
- Are you experiencing *any* mucous buildup symptoms such as a runny nose or sinusitis?
- Do you have any allergy symptoms?
- Are you experiencing asthma, need to clear your throat often or breathing difficulties?
- Do you have reflux?
- Has you skin experienced an outbreak or pimples?
- Are you craving foods and wanting to eat more than before?

INTRODUCTION OF WHEAT & GLUTEN GRAINS: DAY 25-27

Select one wheat—wheat cereal, pasta or barley—item to add back into your diet (i.e., toast, pasta or cooked barley). Start by introducing a serving of grains back into your day with other foods or alone. Over the next three days you can add up to two serving of grains into the day.

In your Reintroducing Foods Journal, answer the following questions each time you eat a food you are reintroducing to your diet.

- Does your body feel different now?
- How does your body feel three hours after eating the reintroduced food?
- How does your body feel one day after eating the reintroduced food?
- How does your body feel three days after eating the reintroduced food?
- Are you bloated, gassy, tired or foggy-headed? Are you experiencing any digestive symptoms?
- Do you have gas or are you bloating?
- Do you have diarrhea?
- Do you have constipation?
- Are you experiencing *any* mucous buildup symptoms such as a runny nose or sinusitis?
- Do you have any allergy symptoms?
- Are you experiencing asthma or breathing difficulties?
- Do you have reflux?
- Has you skin experienced an outbreak or pimples?
- Are you craving foods and wanting to eat more than before?
- Are you experiencing *any* joint pain, discomfort, rashes or general puffiness?
- Are you experiencing an increased appetite to the point of craving after eating?
- Are you experiencing more emotional upsets, a change in emotional state or depressive symptoms?

INTRODUCTION OF COFFEE: DAY 28-30

Start by introducing a cup of coffee in the morning. If you were a coffee addict, you will probably find that one cup of coffee may be all you need now. This is a good thing. You will want to keep your coffee consumption to one cup or less a day per day. Yes, for you hardcore addicts, you may keep it in! However, you may find it doesn't *feel* as good as you remember. Or that you can get by with a lot less!

In your Reintroducing Foods Journal, answer the following questions each time you eat a food you are reintroducing to your diet.

- Does your body feel different now?
- How does your body feel three hours after eating the reintroduced food?
- How does your body feel one day after eating the reintroduced food?
- How does your body feel three days after eating the reintroduced food?
- Are you experiencing any digestive complaints?
- Are you experiencing bloating, gassy feelings or fatigue?
- Are you experiencing diarrhea?
- Are you experiencing constipation?
- Are you experiencing stomach pains after eating?
- Are you experiencing anxiety, nervousness, shaking or tension?
- Do you crave sugar or feel like you are on an emotional rollercoaster?

INTRODUCTION OF HIGH-GLYCEMIC AND CITRUS FRUIT: DAY 31-33

Start by introducing a piece of citrus fruit or a high-sugar fruit such as pineapple, banana or orange. Over the next three days you can add up to two servings of fruit into the day. Eat servings of the fruit for at least 3 days.

In your Reintroducing Foods Journal, answer the following questions each time you eat a food you are reintroducing to your diet.

- Does your body feel different now?
- How does your body feel three hours after eating the reintroduced food?
- How does your body feel one day after eating the reintroduced food?
- How does your body feel three days after eating the reintroduced food?
- Are you experiencing any digestive complaints?

- Are you experiencing bloating, gassy feelings or fatigue?
- Are you experiencing diarrhea?
- Are you experiencing constipation?
- Are you experiencing stomach pains after eating?
- Are you experiencing anxiety, nervousness, shaking or tension?
- Do you crave sugar or feel like you are on an emotional rollercoaster?
- Do you get sores or blisters in you mouth or mucous membrane of the nose?

INTRODUCTION OF SOY: DAY 34-36

Select soy, tofu or tempeh. I am not a fan of drinking of soymilk daily as a substitute for dairy, so if you use soymilk, limit your intake. If you do not eat soy foods, then skip ahead. Start by introducing a serving of soy back into your day with other foods or alone. Over the next three days, you can add up to one serving of soy into the day.

In your Reintroducing Foods Journal, answer the following questions each time you eat a food you are reintroducing to your diet.

- Does your body feel different now?
- How does your body feel three hours after eating the reintroduced food?
- How does your body feel one day after eating the reintroduced food?
- How does your body feel three days after eating the reintroduced food?
- Are you experiencing any digestive complaints?
- Are you experiencing bloating, gassy feelings or fatigue?
- Are you experiencing diarrhea?
- Are you experiencing constipation?
- Are you experiencing stomach pains after eating?
- Are you experiencing anxiety, nervousness, shaking or tension?
- Do you crave sugar or feel like you are on an emotional rollercoaster?
- Are you experiencing *any* mucous buildup symptoms such as a runny nose or sinusitis?
- Are you experiencing allergy symptoms?

- Are you experiencing asthma or breathing difficulties?
- Are you experiencing reflux?
- Has you skin experienced an outbreak or pimples?

INTRODUCTION OF CORN: DAY 37-39

Select corn in its natural form rather than in the form of cornmeal or corn chips. You may add up to two servings a day of corn over the next three days to determine any symptoms. Start by introducing a serving of corn back into your day with other foods or alone. Eat a serving of corn fresh, frozen or from corn meal. Over the next three days you can add up to one serving of corn into the day.

In your Reintroducing Foods Journal, answer the following questions each time you eat a food you are reintroducing to your diet.

- Does your body feel different now?
- How does your body feel three hours after eating the reintroduced food?
- How does your body feel one day after eating the reintroduced food?
- How does your body feel three days after eating the reintroduced food?
- Are you experiencing any digestive complaints?
- Are you experiencing bloating, gassy feelings or fatigue?
- Are you experiencing diarrhea?
- Are you experiencing constipation?
- Are you experiencing stomach pains after eating?
- Are you experiencing anxiety, nervousness, shaking or tension?
- Do you crave sugar or feel like you are on an emotional rollercoaster?
- Are you experiencing *any* mucous buildup symptoms such as a runny nose or sinusitis?
- Are you experiencing allergy symptoms?
- Are you experiencing asthma or breathing difficulties?
- Are you experiencing reflux?
- Has you skin experienced an outbreak or pimples?

INTRODUCTION OF ACIDIC LEGUMES: DAY 40-42

Select a choice of beans: pinto, white beans or kidney beans. These are the more acidic beans we removed form your diet. If you do not eat these types of food, then proceed to next food. Start by introducing a serving of beans back into your day with other foods or alone. Over the next three days you can add up to 1 serving of beans into the day.

In your Reintroducing Foods Journal, answer the following questions each time you eat a food you are reintroducing to your diet.

- Does your body feel different now?
- How does your body feel three hours after eating the reintroduced food?
- How does your body feel one day after eating the reintroduced food?
- How does your body feel three days after eating the reintroduced food?
- Are you experiencing any digestive complaints?
- Are you experiencing bloating, gassy feelings or fatigue?
- Are you experiencing diarrhea?
- Are you experiencing constipation?
- Are you experiencing stomach pains after eating?
- Did you gain weight? Beans have an insulinogenic effect increasing insulin levels over several hours, which may impede weight loss if your insulin management system is off-kilter.

INTRODUCTION OF ALCOHOL (WINE, BEER AND LIQUOR): DAY 43-45

Alcohol is not a food substance. It is not needed or necessary in the human diet. If you do not drink alcohol, please skip this part. Remember small amounts of wine and alcohol have shown to be beneficial; however, alcohol is a toxin and can halt weight loss efforts. Stick with non more than 1 drink a day for a woman and 2 drinks for a man. You may find that you feel the effects—the detoxification efforts of the liver—more readily than you have in the past. You need to be midful of the alcohol you drink. If you drink, drink responsibly.

FOODS YOU SHOULD NOT REINTRODUCE

Food additives, trans-fats, genetically-modified foods, fast foods, high fructose corn syrup (HFCS)processed fructose, excessive alcohol and fake sweeteners should not be reintroduced into the diet. These frankenfoods are not something you need to be putting in your body at all! So, you would do well to never reintroduce these items into your diet.

White, processed and devoid of nutrient foods should be considered a treat and not a requirement in your daily diet. It has only been in the last 50 years that Americans have become the fatest and sickest country due, in a large part, to our diet full of white foods. If someone born in 1900 wouldn't recognize it is food, you shouldn't eat it. Yes, they had dessert but they did not eat mashmallow puff, cream chocolate, nuttry, crunchy, caramel surprise, heart-attack in a plastic bag as a daily snack. The more you reduce, eliminate or keep these foods out of your diet the healthier you will be.

I hope that this program has helped you experience just how powerful our diet is to our physical, mental and emotional wellness. You may have found that certain foods are detracting from your health. Now that you are armed with that knowledge, you are able to keep them out of your diet to keep your symptoms at bay. I know firsthand how foods affect health; I have been gluten-free for years now, and my health has never been better. Knowledge is power. Put that knowledge to work for you.

POST CLEANSE CONSIDERATIONS

- You have control over what you eat, choose wisely. Eat your foods as fresh and organic as possible. The quantity of water that you drink will have a profound impact on your health. Please be sure to drink enough pure water.
- There is no substitute for a daily dose of sunlight, fresh air, exercise and a good night's sleep.
- An awareness of the experience of eating paired with an expression of gratitude for what you are eating will help increase nutritional intuition.
- We were meant to move and exercise often. So, move in a way that moves you!

You made it. I am so happy to have been a part of your journey to a healthier body, mind and spirit. You are now armed to be able to do The Cleanse. May you be well, happy and whole!

References

COFFEE:

http://www.pslgroup.com/dg/eaa4e.htm

http://www.ncbi.nkm.nih.gov/pubmed/2927749

Lynge, E. Anntila, A. and Hemminiki, K. 1997. Organic solvents and cancer. Cancer Causes and Control. 8(3): 406-19.

Liteplo, R.G., Long, G.W. and Meek, M.E. 1998. Relevance of carcinogenicity bioassays in mice in assessing potential health risks associated with exposure to methylene chloride. Human and Experimental Toxicology, 17(2): 84-7.

National Cancer Institute website: http://epi.grants.cancer.gov/. January 2004.

Page, B.D. and Charbonneau, C.F. 1984. Headspace gas chromatographic determination of methylene chloride in decaffeinated tea and coffee, with electrolyte conductivity detection. Journal of the Association of Official Analytical Chemists, 67(4): 757-61.

Cherniske, S. 1998. Caffeine Blues. Warner Books, New York.

McCusker, R.R., Goldberger, B.A. and Cone, E.J. 2003. Caffeine content of specialty coffees. Journal of Analytical Toxicology. 27(7):520-2.

Cherniske, S. 1998. Caffeine Blues. Warner Books, New York.

Feldman, E.J., Isenberg, J.I. and Grossman, M.I. 1981. Gastric acid and gastrin response to decaffeinated coffee and a peptone meal. JAMA. 246(3):248-50.

Cohen, S. and Booth, G.H. Jr. 1975. Gastric acid secretion and lower-esophageal-sphincter pressure in response to coffee and caffeine. New England Journal of Medicine, 293(18):897-9.

Corti, R., Binggeli, C., Sudano, I., Spieker, L, Hanseler, E., Ruschitzka, F., Chaplin, W.F., Luscher, T.F., and Noll, G. 2002. Coffee acutely increases sympathetic nerve activity and blood pressure independently of caffeine content. Role of habitual versus nonhabitual drinking. Circulation. 106:2935-2940.

CORN:

Pollan, Michael (2006), *The Omnivore's Dilemma: A Natural History of Four Meals* Penguin Press, New Your, New York 10014.

DAIRY:

J Paronen, M Knip, E Savilahti, SM Virtanen, J Ilonen, HK Akerblom, O Vaarala. Effect of cow's milk exposure and maternal type 1 diabetes on cellular and humoral immunization to dietary insulin in infants at genetic risk for type 1 diabetes. Diabetes, 2000, Vol 49, Iss 10, pp 1657-1665 Address Paronen J, Natl Publ Hlth Inst, Dept Biochem, Mannerheimintie 166, SF-00300 Helsinki, FINLAND.

Does Dairy Cause Acne?: Canadian Dermatologist Reports Dairy Linked to Acne, http://cookingresources.suite101.com/article.cfm/does_dairy_cause_acne#ixzz0ZDCfKDJr

Campbell, PhD, T. C., The China Study: Startling Implications for Diet, Weight Loss and Health. (BenBella Books; ISBN: 9781932100662), May, 2008.

EXCITOTOXINS:

Blalock, MD, Russell (1997) Excitotoxins, the taste that kills. Health Press NA, Inc. Albuquerque, NM p XVii

http://www.springerlink.com/content/9wk64846k6j871w3/

Wednesday, August 02, 2006. Accessed February 15, 2008

FOOD CLAIMS:

Smith, Jeffrey. (2007) *Genetic Roulette: The Documented Health Risks of Genetically Engineered Foods.* Chelsea Green, White River Junction, Vermont 05001.

Smith, Jeffrey. (2003) *Seeds of Deceptions.* Yes Books, Fairfield, Iowa 52556.

Charles M Benbrook, BioTech InfoNet, Technical Paper Number 6, November 2003

Mexico confirms GM maize contamination' on the Science and Development Network website www.scidev.net/news

Tom Wiley, a farmer in North Dakota, quoted in Seeds of doubt: North American farmers' experiences of GM crops by Hugh Warwick and Gundula Meziani (Soil Association, 2002)

PLASTIC PROBLEMS:

Bisphenol A: Toxic Plastics Chemical in Canned Food. http://www.ewg.org/reports/bisphenola

New Data from CDC Confirms Human Exposure to Bisphenol A in the United States is Far Below Safe Limits." http://www.bisphenol-a.org/whatsNew.

Richter, C.R., Birnbaum, L.S., Farabollini, F., Newbold, R.R., Rubin, B.S., Talsness, C.E., Vandenbergh, J.G., Walser-Kuntz, D.R. and vom Saal, F.S. "In vivo effects of bisphenol A in laboratory rodent studies." Reprod. Toxicol. 24:199-224, 2007.

Shotyk, W., Krachler, M., Chen, B. (2006). Contamination of Canadian and European bottled waters with antimony from PET containers. J. Environ. Monit., 8:288–292.

http://www.rsc.org/publishing/journals/EM/article.asp?doi=b517844b)

Bornehag, C-G., et al., (2004) The Association between Asthma

and Allergic Symptoms in Children and Phthalates in House Dust: A Nested Case-Control Study. Environ. Health Perspect.,

112(14):1393-1397.

http://www.ehponline.org/members/2004/7187/7187.html).

http://www.eurlex.europa.eu/LexUriServ/LexUriServ.do?uri=OJ:L2005:344:0040:0043:EN:PDF)

Ohyama, K., etal. (2001). Certain Styrene Oligomers Have Proliferative Activity on MCF-7 Human Breast Tumor Cells and Binding Affinity for Human Estrogen(http://www.ehponline.org/members/2001/109p699-703ohyama/ohyama-full.html)

Nagel, S.C., vomSaal, F.S., Thayer, K.A., Dhar, M.G., Boechler, M. and Welshons, W.V. (1997).

Relative binding affinity serum modified access (RBASMA) assay predicts the relative in vivo bioactivity of the xenoestrogens bisphenol A and octylphenol. Environ. Health Perspect. 105:70-76.

http://www.pubmedcentral.nih.gov/articlerender.fcgi?artid=1469837).

http://endocrinedisruptors.missouri.edu/vomsaal/vomsaalpubs.html.

http://www.ourstolenfuture.org/newscience/oncompounds/bisphenla/2006/2006-0101vomsaalandwelshons/2006-0101vomsaaland welshons.html.

SOY:

Daniel, Kaayla T. (2004) *The Whole Soy Story: The Dark Side of America's Favorite Health Food.* New Trends Publishing, Inc. Washington, DC 20007.

SUPPLEMENTATION:

Brenna JT. Efficiency of conversion of alpha-linolenic acid to long-chain n-3 fatty acids in man. Curr Opin Clin Nutr Metab Care, 2002. 5:127-132.

Inger Lauritzen, Nicolas Blondeau, Catherine Heurteaux, Catherine Widmann, Georges Romey and Michel Lazdunski (2000). "Polyunsaturated fatty acids are potent neuroprotectors". The EMBO Journal 19 (8): 1784-1793.

Cambridge Applied Polymers Ltd. (04 April 2006). Latest Publications on the Link between DHA and Intelligence / The Brain.

http://www.ehjournal.net/content/4/1/25: Increasing work-place healthiness with the probiotic Lactobacillus reuteri: A randomised, double-blind placebo-controlled study.

SUGAR:

Duffy, William, (1975) Sugar Blues. Time Warner Books. Padnor, PA, 17089

Bhargava, Alok and Amialchuk, Aliaksandr (2007) Added Sugars Displaced the Use of Vital Nutrients in the National Food Stamp Program Survey. http://jn.nutrition.org/cgi/content/abstract/137/2/453 *Why Buy Local: Rise in Ethanol Raises Concerns about Corn as a Food* (January 5, 2007)

My Year of Vegetables (May 27, 2007)

The Cleanse Recipes Shopping List

Meats

- Lean chicken, turkey
- Fish - salmon, halibut, cod, mackerel, tilapia
- Lean red meats
- buffalo, game meat

Fats

- Raw nuts & seeds (not peanuts)
- Freshly ground flaxseed meal
- Olive oil, olives
- Almonds
- Cashews
- Pine Nuts
- Sunflower Seeds
- Flaxseed oil
- Avocado
- Butter
- Coconut milk
- Coconut oil

Non-starchy vegetables

- Arugula

- Asparagus
- Beet greens
- Bell peppers (red, yellow, green)
- All peppers
- Broccoli
- Brussels sprouts
- Cabbage
- Cauliflower
- Celery
- Chives
- Collard greens
- Cucumber
- Dandelion greens
- Eggplant
- Garlic
- Ginger root
- Green beans
- Jicama (raw)
- Jalapeno peppers
- Kale
- Lettuce
- Mustard greens
- Onions
- Parsley
- Radish
- Snap beans
- Snow peas
- Shallots

- Spinach
- Spaghetti squash
- Summer squash
- Swiss chard
- Tomatoes
- Watercress

Starchy Carbohydrate Choices

- Winter squash
- Artichokes
- Leeks
- Okra
- Pumpkin
- Sweet potato or yam
- Turnip
- Chick peas (garbanzo)
- Millet
- Quinoa
- Amaranth
- Black beans
- Lentils and Mung bean

Fruits

- Berries (blackberries, blueberries, boysenberries, elderberries, gooseberries, loganberries, raspberries, strawberries)
- Pear
- Apples
- Lemons
- Limes
- Grapefruit

- Orange

Spices

- Black pepper
- Chili pepper flakes
- Chili powder
- Fresh Cilantro
- Cinnamon
- Cocoa powder
- Ginger
- Herbs de Provence
- Fresh Mint
- Mustard powder
- Oregano
- Paprika
- Fresh or dried parsley
- Fresh or dried sage
- Sea Salt
- Tarragon
- Really any spices will do just fine!

Sauces and Nut Butters

- Chili in Adobo Sauce
- Fish Sauce (Asian section of market)
- Tahini – sesame butter
- Ume Plum Vinegar (Asian section of market)
- Almond, cashew or macadamia butter

Sweeteners

Stevia and/or Xylitol

The Cleanse Basic Recipes

Shakes and Smoothies

BASIC SHAKE

- 2 scoops The Cleanse Detox Formula
- 6 oz. ice
- 8 oz. water

Instructions

Blend in a blender until creamy and smooth

Variations:

- ½ cup frozen berries
- 1-3 tablespoon freshly-ground flaxseed meal (makes shake thick)
- 1 teaspoon no sugar added vanilla extract
- 1-2 teaspoon Xylitol powder or Stevia
- Replace water with unsweetened coconut milk or flavored almond milk.

BASIC FRUIT SHAKE

- 2 scoops The Cleanse Detox Formula
- 8 oz. frozen cleanse fruit choices
- 8 oz. water or almond milk or rice milk

Instructions

Blend in a blender until creamy and smooth

Variations:

- 1-3 tablespoon freshly-ground flaxseed meal (makes shake thick)
- 1 teaspoon no sugar added vanilla extract
- 1-2 teaspoon Xylitol powder or Stevia
- Replace water with unsweetened coconut milk or flavored almond milk.

BASIC ALMOND BUTTER SHAKE

- 2 scoops tablespoons almond butter
- 6 oz. ice
- 8 oz. almond or rice milk

Instructions

Blend in a blender until creamy and smooth

GREAT GUT PUDDING SMOOTHIE

- 1 cup organic unsweetened applesauce
- 1-3 tablespoons freshly ground flaxseed meal
- 1 scoop Cleanse Detox Formula
- 1 tablespoon Glutamine powder
- 1 tablespoon Almond or Cashew butter
- ½ to 1 teaspoon Xylitol or Stevia

Instructions

Blend in a blender until creamy and smooth

POWER MILLET OR QUINOA SHAKE

- 1 cup cooked millet cold or other long-cooking whole grain cereal
- ¼ cup blueberries
- 1-2 teaspoon Xylitol powder or Stevia
- 1 tablespoon chopped nuts

Instructions

After cooking and cooling, blend in a blender until creamy and smooth

Then add 1 scoop Cleanse Detox Formula and 1 teaspoon Xylitol powder and top with 1 tablespoon chopped nuts

BERRY COMPOTE

Warm up 1 cup frozen berries

Top with this mixture: 1 scoop Cleanse Detox Formula mixed in ¼ coconut milk, 1 teaspoon Xylitol powder, and 1 tablespoon raw chopped nuts.

Breakfast foods

CHICKEN BREAKFAST SAUSAGES

- 2 oz. Ground chicken or Turkey breast
- ½ cup chopped spinach
- Pinch of dill and sage herbs

Instructions

- Mix together and sauté.
- Serve with Tomato or avocado slices

MORNING NO-OAT MEAL

- 1 cup cooked millet, quinoa or other long-cooking whole grain (use leftover) or 1/2 cup quinoa flakes, or rice meal with 1 cup water prepared
- 1 teaspoon Xylitol
- 1 tablespoon chopped nuts
- 1 teaspoon coconut oil
- ¼ cup berries or cut apple or ½ cup applesauce

Instructions

If using precooked grains, heat 1/2 cup cooked grain in pan with 2 tablespoons of water. If making quinoa flakes or rice meal breakfast cereal, follow directions on the box.

Then add 1 scoop Cleanse Detox Formula, 1/2 cup berries or cut apple or 1/2 cup applesauce and 1 teaspoon Xylitol powder and top with 1 tablespoon chopped nuts.

CINNAMON BAKED SQUASH

- 1 medium squash
- 1 tablespoon cinnamon
- 1-2 tablespoons xylitol or stevia
- **Instructions**

Wash and cut squash in half. Take seeds out. Put squash in a baking dish, add your choice of sweetener, and sprinkle with cinnamon. Bake them for 45 minutes at 450 degrees. Squash is often sweet enough. You can omit the sweeteners, or use apple chunks. You can save the seeds and soak and bake them.

POTATO PANCAKES

I like to serve them with fresh applesauce.

- 3 large sweet potatoes (about 2 pounds)
- 1 large sweet onion
- 1 cup Ground quinoa or flax meal (½ cup in pancakes, ½ cup used to coat the outside of the pancake)
- 1 tablespoon olive oil
- 1 teaspoon salt, or more to taste
- ¼ cup coconut oil

Instructions

Blend in a blender until creamy and smooth. Preheat oven to 425 degrees. Clean sweet potatoes and bake until fork done (you can use leftover sweet potatoes). Remove from oven, mix all ingredients except for coconut oil. Make patties and coat outside with ground quinoa or flax meal. Sauté in coconut oil. Serve with applesauce and cinnamon.

AMARANTH OR QUINOA PUDDING

- 2 cups amaranth or quinoa, cooked
- ½ cup almonds, chopped fine
- 1- 2 tsp Xylitol nectar
- juice of ½ lemon
- 1 cup water
- 1 ½ teaspoon vanilla
- grated rind of one lemon
- dash of cinnamon

Instructions

Combine ingredients in a large sauce pan, cover and bring to a boil. Reduce heat and simmer for 15 minutes. Pour pudding into individual dessert bowls. Top with a few strawberries and chill.

QUINOA PORRIDGE

- ½ cup quinoa cooked
- ½ cup berries
- 1 teaspoon butter or coconut butter
- Cinnamon to taste

Instructions

Combine ingredients in a large sauce pan, cover and bring to a boil. Reduce heat and simmer for 15 minutes.

- Toasted almonds optional
- 2 tsp Xylitol

OTHER BREAKFAST OPTIONS:

- Leftovers from last night's dinner
- Vegetable soups
- Green Smoothie from the advance recipes

Soups

MEDITERRANEAN GRILLED VEGETABLE SOUP

- 1 yellow bell pepper, seeded and quartered
- 2 small zucchini, seeded and quartered
- ¼ cup shredded basil leaves
- ½ tablespoon distilled vinegar
- salt & freshly ground black pepper to taste.
- 1 red onion, quartered
- 1 teaspoon olive oil
- 3 large tomatoes chopped or canned diced tomato
- 1 clove garlic, peeled
- ½ teaspoon dried oregano

Instructions

Prepare a grill or preheat the broiler. Grill or broil bell peppers, skin-side toward the flame, until the skin is blackened, 5 to 10 minutes. Place in a paper bag and set aside for 15 minutes.

Meanwhile, brush zucchini and onion slices with oil and grill or broil until well browned and tender, about 5 minutes. Chop coarsely and set aside.

Peel the peppers. Coarsely chop the yellow pepper and set aside with the reserved zucchini and onions. Place the red peppers in a food processor or blender, along with tomatoes, garlic and oregano; puree until smooth. Transfer to a bowl and stir in 1 cup water, basil, distilled vinegar and the reserved chopped vegetables. Season with salt and pepper. Cover and refrigerate until cool, about 30 minutes. (The soup can be stored, covered, in the refrigerator for up to 2 days.)

GINGER & SWEET POTATO SOUP WITH CILANTRO

- 2 teaspoons olive oil
- 1 medium carrot, chopped
- 2 cups diced sweet potato
- 1 medium leek, white part only, cut in half lengthwise, rinsed well between layers and thinly sliced

- 1 1-inch piece fresh ginger, peeled and finely chopped, plus 1 teaspoon grated
- ¾ teaspoon salt, or to taste
- 4 cups chicken broth, homemade or canned in a pinch, or vegetable stock
- Fresh cilantro leaves for garnish

Instructions

Heat oil in a 4- to 6-quart Dutch oven or soup pot over medium-high heat. Add leek and carrot; cook, stirring often, until they begin to soften, 2 to 3 minutes. Stir in sweet potatoes (or yams) and chopped ginger. Add broth and bring to a boil. Cover, reduce heat to low and simmer until sweet potatoes are soft, about 30 minutes.

In batches, if necessary, transfer the soup to a blender or food processor and process until smooth. Return the soup to the pot, season with salt and reheat. Just before serving, stir in grated ginger. Ladle soup into bowls. Draw the tip of a knife or a toothpick through the yogurt to make decorative swirls. Garnish with cilantro and serve with lime wedges.

VEGETABLE SOUP

- ¼ cup sliced celery
- 2 tablespoon diced onion
- 1 garlic cloves, minced
- 1 cups fat free broth
- ½ cup diced green or red cabbage
- ¼ cup green beans
- 1 teaspoon tomato paste
- ¼ teaspoon basil
- pinch of oregano
- dash of salt
- ¼ cup zucchini

Instructions

Place all the ingredients in a pot. Bring to boil, then reduce the heat and simmer until the vegetables are tender. Makes 2-3 cups of soup.

KHICHADI RECIPE

Khichadi is a simple, easily digested stew traditionally used in Auyveda during a cleanse. I have updated it here with some small tweaks.

- ½ cup brown basmati rice, soaked for at least ½ hour and drained
- ½ cup mung beans or lentils, soaked in water for at least 1 hour and drained
- 2 tablespoons ghee or clarified butter
- ½ 1 teaspoon cumin
- ½ medium onion, finely chopped
- ½ teaspoon chopped ginger
- 1 cup vegetables, such as peas, chopped kale, spinach
- 4 cups vegetable stock, chicken stock (advanced recipes or store bought)
- 1 teaspoon garlic sautéed until golden brown
- 1 teaspoon of turmeric powder
- ¼ teaspoon of black pepper
- 1 bay leaf

Instructions

Heat ghee (clarified butter) or olive oil in a pan over moderate heat. Add cumin or coriander seeds. Then add finely chopped, medium onion, chopped ginger and garlic; sauté until golden brown. Stir in turmeric powder, black pepper and 1 bay leaf. Add mung beans, water, vegetables, and rice. Cook for about an hour. When the beans are completely soft, add a pinch of salt. Serve this dish with ghee and chopped fresh cliantro leaves.

SPRING SAVORY SOUP

- 12 stalks medium asparagus (or 17 thin stalks)
- 1 avocado
- 5-6 tomatoes
- 1 cup fresh curly parsley
- 3-5 sun-dried tomatoes (bottled in olive oil) or dry
- ¼ cup dried onion
- 4 cloves fresh garlic
- 1 red bell pepper
- Sea salt to taste
- 2 teaspoon Dill
- 2 lime, cut in thin slices

Instructions

Trim and dice the tips from the asparagus and set aside for a garnish. In a food processor or blender, blend the asparagus and red tomatoes, parsley, dried tomatoes, spices, garlic, onion and red bell pepper. Then blend the avocado until soup is smooth and creamy. Warm in a skillet and garnish with lemon or lime slices on top. Season with sea salt to taste or serve cold in the summertime. Sprinkle diced asparagus tips on top just before serving. Yummy!

CURRY-TASTIC SOUP

- 1-2 cups broccoli, chopped
- 1-2 cups cauliflower, chopped
- 1 cup Jerusalem artichokes chopped
- 1 cup veggie broth
- 1 avocado
- 1 clove garlic, minced
- ¼ teaspoon curry powder
- 1 Tablespoon lemon or lime juice
- ½ teaspoon sea salt

Instructions

In a food processor or blender, combine the avocado with the veggie broth or broth, and garlic. Blend well. With machine still running, add the broccoli and cauliflower and blend until smooth. Lastly blend in seasonings and lemon/lime juice and salt. Add more broth or water to desired consistency. Warm on the stove in a sauce pan.

CHUNK-ASTIC VEGGIE SOUP

- 2 ½ cups tomato juice (canned or fresh)
- 1 avocado
- 6-8 celery stalks
- 2 carrots
- 1 summer squash
- 1 bunch of spinach or arugula
- 3 leaves of fresh basil
- 1 teaspoon coriander

Instructions

For broth, blend tomato juice, avocado and 3-4 celery stalks. Grate squash and carrots and celery, adding finely chopped arugula and other fresh green spices last. Serve in a bowl or cup; decorate with fresh herbs. Warm on the stove in a sauce pan.

CREAMY BROCCOLI SOUP

- 2 cups vegetable stock or chicken stock
- 3-4 cups broccoli, chopped
- 1 red bell pepper or yellow, chopped
- 2 red or yellow onions, chopped
- 1 avocado
- 1-2 stalks celery, cut in large pieces
- Salt and pepper to taste
- cumin and ginger to taste

Instructions

In an pot, warm 2 cups of water or stock add the chopped broccoli and warm for 5 minutes. In a blender, puree the warmed broccoli, bell pepper, onion, avocado, and celery, thinning with additional water as necessary to achieve the desired consistency. Serve warm, flavoring with fresh ginger, cumin or any other spices you like. Add a slice of lemon on top to garnish.

TOMATO CREAM SOUP

- 4 Roma tomatoes
- 2 green onion tips (about 1 inch of white/light green part)
- ¼ green pepper
- 1 cup vegetable broth
- 1 avocado
- 1 teaspoon sea salt
- pepper to taste

Instructions

Add all ingredients and liquefy in blender. Heat just to warm

THAI PUMPKIN SOUP

- 1 tablespoon vegetable oil
- 1 tablespoon butter
- 1 clove garlic, chopped
- 1 tablespoon chopped lemon grass (optional)
- 2 cups chicken stock
- 4 shallots, chopped (1/2 onion can be used as a substitute)
- 2 fresh red chili peppers, chopped
- 4 cups peeled and diced pumpkin
- 1 ½ cups coconut milk
- 1 bunch fresh basil leaves

Instructions

In a medium saucepan, heat oil and butter over low heat. Cook garlic, shallots, chilies, and lemongrass in oil until fragrant (be careful not to burn the garlic). Stir in chicken stock, coconut milk, and pumpkin; bring to a boil. Cook until pumpkin softens. In a blender, blend the soup in batches to a smooth or slightly chunky consistency, whatever you prefer. Serve with basil leaves.

BUTTERNUT SQUASH SOUP

- 2 tablespoons ghee, butter, or olive oil
- 1 small onion, chopped (1/2 cup)
- 2 cups vegetable or chicken broth
- 1 teaspoon minced fresh ginger
- 1/4 teaspoon sea salt
- 1/4 teaspoon white pepper
- 1/4 teaspoon ground coriander
- 1 pound butternut squash, peeled, seeded, and cut into 1-inch cubes
- 2 medium pears, peeled and sliced
- 1 tablespoon chopped fresh rosemary
- 1/4 teaspoon ground cinnamon
- 1 cup almond milk
- 1/2 cup chopped toasted pecans, for garnish

Instructions

Melt ghee in a large pot over medium heat. Cook onion in ghee, stirring occasionally, until tender. Stir in broth, squash, two sliced pears, rosemary, ginger, and remaining spices. Heat to boiling; reduce heat. Cover and simmer 10–15 minutes or until squash is fork tender. Purée soup in batches in food processor or blender. Return puréed soup to pot. Stir in almond milk. Reheat, stirring frequently, until hot (do not boil). Garnish with pecans and sliced pear.

BEAN AND ASPARAGUS SOUP

- 2 carrots, shaved
- 2 celery stalks, cut as desired
- 6 sprigs of parsley
- 1 onion, chopped
- 4 cups water
- 2 cups crisp-steamed green beans
- 1 1/2 cups crisp-steamed asparagus
- 1 Teaspoon of basil
- 1 bay leaf
- 1 teaspoon sea salt

Instructions

Chop all vegetable ingredients in food processor and add to 4 cups of water or Vegetable stock in a soup pot. Lightly simmer until vegetables are just softened- about 8-10 minutes-then out contents into a blender and thoroughly puree until thick, creamy texture is achieved. Add salt and seasonings. Serve warm. Optional seasoning suggestions include ½ teaspoon cumin, ½ teaspoon dill, ½ teaspoon herbs de Provence.

SPINACH SOUP

- 1 avocado
- 1 cucumber
- 2 green onions
- 1 clove garlic
- ¼ red bell pepper
- 1 cup water or vegetable stock
- 2 cups fresh raw spinach
- Sea salt to taste
- 1 teaspoon curry powder
- fresh lime juice to taste

Instructions

In a blender, add the avocado and half of the water or stock and puree, then add the rest of the ingredients one at a time, blending to desired thickness and thinning with the remaining water if desired. Add salt to taste, and flavor with spices and lime juice to your desire.

VEGETABLE MINESTRONE SOUP

- 1 small cabbage
- 1 onion
- 2 celery
- 1 zucchini
- 1 red bell pepper
- 2 carrots
- 1 yellow squash

Instructions

Cut vegetables as preferred. Cover carrots and celery with water in soup pot. Cook gently until they just begin to "give", then add remaining ingredients. Do not overcook. Serve hot with olive oil, sea salt and cayenne pepper to taste.

ADUKI BEANS SOUP

- 8 ounces dry aduki beans
- 6 cups water
- 1 bay leaf
- 1 clove garlic, finely minced
- 1 teaspoon ground allspice
- 1 large onion, finely chopped
- 4 stalks celery, thinly sliced
- 3 cloves
- 2 teaspoons salt
- 3 teaspoons white pepper

Instructions

Wash the aduki beans well in several changes of water, then drain. In a large pot, bring the 6 cups water to a boil. Add all ingredients and boil rapidly for 15 minutes. Reduce heat and simmer, covered, for 2 hours. You may puree fully or partially for a smoother soup, but I prefer it just as it is.

LENTIL SOUP

- 1 teaspoon olive oil
- 2 tablespoon carrot, finely chopped
- 2 cups chicken or vegetable stock
- 2 tablespoon onion, finely chopped
- 1 small sprig fresh thyme or 1/4 teaspoon dried
- 2/3 cup dried lentils
- salt and pepper to taste

Instructions

Heat the olive oil in a saucepan over low heat. Add the carrot, celery, onion and thyme, season lightly with pepper and cook for 10 minutes. (Do not add salt until the lentils are fully cooked, because salt will prevent the lentils from becoming tender.) Add the stock and lentils, and bring to a boil quickly over high heat. Lower the heat and simmer until the lentils are tender, about 1 hour. Puree 2/3 of the soup in a blender and stir it into the remaining 1/3. If the soup is too thick, thin it by adding a little more stock. Raise the heat and bring the soup to a boil for 15 seconds.

Salads

ASIAN COLESLAW

Adapted from Institute of Integrative Nutrition Recipe

- 1 medium head green cabbage
- 1 medium head red cabbage
- 3 tablespoons sea salt
- 3 large carrots
- ¼ cup minced scallions
- 1 tablespoon toasted sesame seeds

Dressing:
- 2/3 cup unseasoned Ume plum vinegar
- 2 tbsp Xylitol or 1 tbsp Stevia
- 1 ½ tablespoons dark-roasted sesame oil

Instructions

Discard the outer leaves of cabbage. Cut heads in quarters; remove and discard cores. Slice cabbage thinly or shred in a food processor. Layer the cabbage in a large bowl with the sea salt. Toss to distribute salt evenly and let cabbage sit for 1 hour to soften.

Meanwhile, peel the carrots and grate them into thin shreds.

Drain off any liquid produced by the cabbage and rinse the cabbage well in several changes of cold water to remove excess salt. Taste the cabbage; if it is still too salty, rinse it again.

Add carrots to the cabbage and mix well.

Whisk the ume plum vinegar, Xylitol or Stevia and sesame oil together in a small bowl.

Pour the dressing over the cabbage and mix well. Let chill. Garnish with minced scallions and toasted sesame seeds before serving.

SCRUMPTIOUS SWEET POTATO SALAD

- 1 large peeled sweet potato
- 1 ½ tablespoon olive oil
- Salt and pepper
- 1 large red onion, peeled and cut into about 10 wedges
- 4 medium garlic cloves, unpeeled
- About a handful of topped and tailed green beans
- 1 tablespoon Ume Plum vinegar
- 2 tablespoon mild sweet prepared chili sauce

Instructions

Preheat oven to 375F degrees.

Cut sweet potato into 1/2 inch slices. Cut larger slices in half.

Place sweet potato slices and onion wedges in a single layer on a large baking tray. Drizzle with oil and toss to coat. Season with salt and pepper. Bake for 15 minutes.

Stir potatoes and onions.

Add garlic to the tray. Return tray to oven and cook for a further 20-30 minutes, or until vegetables are tender and onion has lightly caramelized. Turn vegetables once during cooking.

Half fill a medium saucepan with water and bring to the boil. Add beans to saucepan and boil for about 3 minutes, until beans are tender but still a bit crisp. Remove from heat and drain. Place beans in a bowl of cold water for 10 seconds to stop the cooking process. Drain and cut into 3/4 inch lengths.

Squeeze roasted garlic from its skin and place in a small bowl. Mash garlic using a fork. Add ume plum vinegar and chili sauce to garlic and stir to combine.

Toss dressing, beans, sweet potato and onion together in a large bowl. Serve salad hot or cold. Store any leftover salad in an airtight container in the refrigerator.

RAW TABOULI!

- 1 bunch cilantro
- 1 bunch parsley
- 1 bunch green onions
- 2 tomatoes chopped and seeded
- 1 avocado
- ½ cup of raw almonds
- ½ cup cold-pressed olive oil
- 1 teaspoon sea salt
- 1 tbsp Xylitol or 1/2 tbsp Stevia
- ½ lemon

Instructions

Chop up cilantro, parsley, green onions, avocados and tomatoes in a bowl. Blend almonds to a fine flour in blender and add to bowl. Add the juice of half a lemon, a tablespoon of olive oil, a tablespoon of xylitol or stevia, and a teaspoon of salt. Change it up each time by adding a different vegetable/herb like corn, broccoli, or fresh basil, or a different spice like Italian or Mexican seasonings.

ASIAN SUMMER SALAD

Courtesy of Integrative Nutrition

- ½ cup diced celery
- ½ medium cucumber
- 2 large tomatoes
- ½ lemon
- 2 tbsp Xylitol or 1 tbsp Stevia
- 2 tablespoons Ume plum vinegar
- 1/8 teaspoon salt
- minced ginger (to taste)
- lettuce leaves, or greens

Instructions

Chill the celery, cucumber and tomatoes. Dice the celery into small pieces. Dice or slice the cucumber, according to your preference. Dice or slice the tomatoes, according to your preference. Combine the xylitol or stevia, Ume plum vinegar, and salt and mix well. Arrange lettuce leaves or greens on a serving plate. Place celery, cucumbers, and tomatoes on lettuce or greens. Lightly pour dressing over vegetables. Squeeze lemon juice, to taste, over salad. Sprinkle with minced ginger and enjoy!

LUCKY LUCY SALAD

- 3 cups thin sliced cut kale
- 1 ½ cups shredded purple cabbage
- ½ shredded beets
- 2 carrots, grated
- 3 green onions, sliced
- 1 tomato diced
- 2 celery stalks, thinly sliced
- ¼ cup mashed avocado
- 2 teaspoon lemon juice

Instructions

Peel beets and onions. Grate carrots, beets, onion. Thinly slice cabbage, kale and dice tomatoes. Combine the cabbage, beets, carrots, onions, and celery in a large bowl. Add the avocado and lemon juice and toss to mix.

BLACK BEAN, JICAMA AND CARROT SALAD

- 2 15-ounce cans black beans, rinsed, drained
- 1 cup 1/3-inch dice peeled jicama
- 1/3 cup thinly sliced green onions
- 1/3 cup chopped fresh cilantro
- ¼ cup (packed) chopped fresh basil
- 5 tablespoons extra-virgin olive oil, divided
- ½ cup 1/3-inch dice peeled carrots
- 3 tablespoons fresh lime juice
- 2 tablespoons orange juice
- 2 ½ teaspoons grated lime peel
- ¼ teaspoon ground cumin

Instructions

In a bowl add black beans, jicama, carrots, green onions, cilantro, and basil.

Whisk lime juice, orange juice, lime peel, cumin, and remaining 4 tablespoons oil in small bowl. Mix dressing into bean salad. Season generously with salt and pepper. (Can be made 4 hours ahead. Cover; chill. Let stand at room temperature 1 hour before serving.)

SPINACH CAESAR SALAD

- 1 large bunch spinach
- 1-2 garlic cloves, pressed
- ½ lemon, juiced
- ½-1 teaspoon mustard powder
- ½ cup Almond slivers
- 2 tablespoon olive oil (extra virgin)
- pinch of sea salt
- Sprinkle of freshly ground white pepper

Instructions

Rinse the spinach very well under running water. Once clean, spin the spinach leaves dry in a salad spinner and put into a large bowl. Tear or cut leaves into bite-size pieces. Add sesame or slivered almonds.

In a small bowl, blend 1 or 2 pressed cloves of garlic, lemon juice, mustard, olive oil, a sprinkle of white pepper and sea salt. Pour over the spinach and toss well.

KITCHEN SINK SALAD

- 1 red bell pepper chopped
- 1 orange chopped
- juice 2 small limes
- 1 garlic clove crushed
- 1 handful of raw cashews
- 1 yellow, chopped
- 5-6 medium tomatoes chopped
- 2 avocados, diced
- sea salt to taste

Instructions

Toss all ingredients together in large bowl, serve and enjoy!

SUMMER SALAD

- 1 head of romaine lettuce chopped
- 3 red radish chopped
- ¼ red onion chopped
- 1 teaspoon minced garlic
- 2 tablespoon cold pressed flax oil
- 1 avocado, diced
- 3 medium tomatoes
- 1 stalk celery chopped
- 2 red bell peppers, chopped
- Juice of 1 lemon
- sea salt to taste

Instructions

Toss all ingredients together in large bowl, serve and enjoy!

CARROT CRUNCH SALAD

- 1 cup shredded carrots
- 1 cup celery slices
- 1 small red, orange or yellow bell pepper, chopped
- ½ cup raw walnuts, chopped
- sea salt to taste
- juice of 1-2 limes
- 1 tablespoon of olive oil
- 1 tablespoon of almond butter

Instructions

Toss all ingredients together in large bowl, let sit for 5-10 minutes. Enjoy!

SALSA SALAD

- 1 cup black beans rinsed and drained
- ½ cup shredded carrots
- ½ cup celery slices
- 1 large red, yellow, or orange bell pepper, chopped
- 1 cup cucumber, chopped into bite sized chunks
- 1 cup fresh salsa
- ½ cup raw pine nuts or raw cashews
- sea salt to taste

Instructions

In a bowl combine black beans, celery, carrots, peppers, and cucumber. Blend salsa and nuts together to make a creamy dressing. Toss other ingredients together in large bowl, mix in dressing. Enjoy!

CARIBE-BEAN SALAD

- 1 tablespoon olive oil
- 1 ½ tablespoon lime juice
- ½ teaspoon chili powder
- 2 tablespoon shredded carrot

- 2 tablespoon slivered red onion
- 1 cup loose-packed, finely chopped kale leaves
- 15 oz. 1 can black beans, rinsed and drained

Instructions

In a bowl, whisk oil, lime juice, and salt and chili powder to taste. Add beans, kale, carrot and onion. Stir to coat ingredients with dressing.

OLIVE OIL & LIME DRESSING

- 1 cup water
- 2 tablespoon Lime juice
- zest of lime (scrap the green skin with planer)
- 1 cup extra virgin olive oil
- sea salt and black pepper to taste

Instructions

Using a blender or an electric mixing stick; combine purified water, lime juice , extra virgin olive oil and salt. Taste and re-season with lime zest and salt if necessary.

You can add a little xylitol or stevia if necessary to sweeten.

TAHINI DRESSING

- 3 tablespoons olive oil
- 3 cloves garlic, chopped
- fresh black pepper (a couple of dashes)
- juice of 1 lemon
- ½ cup Tahini
- 2 teaspoons Ume plum vinegar (Asian aisle)
- ½ teaspoon paprika
- ¼ cup lightly packed fresh parsley
- ½ cup cold water

Instructions

Add garlic and all ingredients except parsley to the food processor and blend until smooth. Add the parsley and pulse until parsley is very finely chopped but not blended in. Refrigerate at least an hour in an airtight container.

BASIC ITALIAN DRESSING

- 6 tablespoons olive oil
- 2 tablespoons chopped fresh parsley
- 3 tablespoon fresh lemon juice
- 2 garlic cloves, chopped
- 1 teaspoon dried basil, crumbled
- ¼ teaspoon dried crushed red pepper
- Pinch of dried oregano

Instructions

Combine all ingredients in small bowl and whisk to blend.

Season to taste with salt and pepper.

AVOCADO SALAD DRESSING

- 1 ripe avocado
- ¼ cup coconut milk
- ¼ tablespoon garlic powder
- 1 tablespoon fresh lemon juice
- ¼ tablespoon salt
- 1/8 tablespoon black pepper

Instructions

Combine all ingredients in a blender and blend until smooth and creamy.

ITALIAN MUSTARD DRESSING

- 1 teaspoon garlic, minced
- 2 teaspoons shallot, minced (use onion in a pinch)
- ½ teaspoon ground black pepper
- 1 1/3 cups olive oil
- 2 tablespoons mustard powder
- 1 ½ teaspoons dried oregano
- 2 teaspoons dried parsley
- ¼ teaspoon salt
- 3 tablespoon lemon juice

Instructions

Process all the ingredients except the oil in a blender. Slowly blend in oil. Set aside in the refrigerator.

Vegetable Dishes

HOT SPOT GREENS

- 1 bunch broccoli rabe, Swiss chard, kale, mustard greens or spinach
- 2 cloves garlic, minced
- 2 teaspoons coconut oil
- Red hot pepper flakes
- Pinch of salt
- 1 teaspoon of toasted sesame oil (optional)
- 2 tablespoon toasted sesame seeds (optional)

Instructions

Wash the greens well. Chop them into bite-sized pieces. You may want to chop the stems thinner and cook them separately.

In a large skillet heat coconut oil. Add garlic, hot pepper flakes and stems (if desired) and sauté until garlic just begins to turn golden. Add the greens and stir-fry until all the leaves are wilted. Add 1/4 cup water if the pan seems too dry and continue to stir-fry until the greens are done to your liking. Sprinkle with salt, sesame seeds and serve immediately.

SAUTÉED BROCCOLI AND CARROTS

- ½ pound Brussels sprouts
- ½ pound carrots
- olive oil
- salt and pepper

Instructions

Chop broccoli into florets. Peel and chop the stalks. Cut carrots thick on diagonal.

In a pot of boiling water with salt, blanch carrots and broccoli until tender crisp. Sauté vegetables in olive oil. Add salt and pepper to taste. Serve immediately.

STIR-FRYING VEGETABLES

Courtesy of Integrative Nutrition

Stir-frying is another quick, tasty and nutritious way to prepare vegetables. You can stir-fry in either oil or water. Stir-frying in oil makes a tastier dish since the hot oil seals in the flavor and nutrients. Any kind of vegetables can be used. The softer vegetables like Chinese cabbage, bok choy, thinly sliced carrots, mushrooms and onions will only take a few minutes to cook.

Here are some great colorful and tasty combinations:

- onions, carrots and snow peas
- Chinese cabbage, mung bean sprouts and scallions
- leeks, carrots and red peppers
- onions, mushrooms and zucchini with dried basil
- yellow patty pan squash and greens with garlic

Instructions

Before you start, have all of the vegetables cut into desired pieces-thinner slices and smaller pieces will cook faster and more evenly.

Heat a wok or a frying pan and add a small amount of oil. If you are making a small amount of vegetables, usually just brushing the pan with coconut oil is enough. Start with the harder vegetables like roots. Add them one kind at a time and cook them until they become shiny, before adding the next ones. Sprinkling a pinch of salt over the vegetables draws just enough moisture to prevent sticking and it also makes them taste sweeter.

At the end of cooking you can make a nice sauce, thickened with arrowroot or kuzu and seasoned fish sauce, ginger or garlic.

KALE POTATO CHIPS

- 1 bunch Dinosaur (Lactinate) Kale (non-curly leaves)
- ½ tablespoon olive oil
- salt and pepper to taste

Instructions

Heat oven to 350. Trim stalks from Kale. Place leaves in a large bowl, add oil and toss to coat the leaves. Salt and pepper to taste. Bake for 20 minutes. Check to see if leaves are dry. If they still are limp, let them cook up to ten minutes more. Remove from oven and eat.

SAUTÉED CABBAGE AND LEEKS

- 1 tablespoon oil
- 1 tablespoon minced garlic
- ½ head red cabbage, chopped or other green
- 3 leeks, white parts alone, cleaned and sliced

Instructions

Heat oil over medium heat in a skillet until hot. Add cabbage & leeks, saute until just about tender, about 5 to 7 minutes.

Stir in the garlic and continue to sauté until the cabbage and leeks are completely tender, this should only take a further 1 minute or so; be careful not to overcook. Serve immediately.

SIMMERED GREENS WITH ONION

- 1 ¼ lb. collard greens, kale, or chard
- 1 tablespoon organic extra virgin olive oil
- 1 medium onion, minced
- pinch of salt
- ¾ cups vegetable stock

Instructions

Wash the greens and shake them dry. Remove the stems and cut the leaves into large pieces. Heat the oil in a large, heavy saucepan. Add the onion and sauté until it becomes transparent. Stir in the greens. Add salt, and cook for one minute. Pour in the broth, stir and simmer until greens are tender.

SWEET POTATO OVEN FRIES

- 2 ½ pounds sweet potatoes
- 1/3 cup olive salt and freshly ground black pepper

- Salt and freshly ground black pepper
- Optional taste ideas: 1 teaspoon paprika or cayenne pepper or cinnamon

Instructions

Arrange two racks at center and lower positions of the oven, and preheat oven to 400 degrees. Line two rimmed baking sheets with aluminum foil.

Cut sweet potatoes into wedges, and trim stem ends. Put oil and spices in a plastic bag. Put sweet potatoes in bag and shake. Take the potatoes out and arrange on a baking sheet. You may liberally add additional spices to taste. Bake for 30-40 minutes. The outsides should be a little crispy with softer insides. Let cool a little and eat

OVEN ROASTED VEGETABLES

- 1 lb. new potatoes
- 1 lb. yams
- 3 large carrots
- 1 medium onion
- 1 large red pepper
- 1 large green pepper
- 1 bunch radishes (optional)
- 2 tablespoon olive oil
- 1 tablespoon chopped fresh or 1 teaspoon dried thyme
- 1 tablespoon chopped fresh or 1 teaspoon dried oregano

Instructions

Preheat oven to 400 degrees. Cut new potatoes into 1 inch pieces. Peel yams, cut into 1 inch pieces. Cut carrots into 1 inch pieces. Cut onion into 1/2 inch wedges. Cut green and red peppers into 1 inch pieces. Trim edges from radishes. In roasting pan toss vegetables with olive and herbs. Toast 1 hour until vegetables are tender, stirring occasionally.

CINNAMON BAKED SQUASH

- 1 medium squash
- 1 tablespoon cinnamon
- 1-2 xylitol or stevia

Instructions

Wash and cut squash in half. Take seeds out. Put squash in a baking dish, add your choice of sweetener, and sprinkle with cinnamon. Bake them for 45 minutes at 450 degrees.

Often times squashes are sweet enough just by themselves, so you can omit the sweeteners, or use apple chunks.

You can save the seeds and soak and bake them.

DANDELION GREENS

- 1 pound dandelion greens
- ½ cup chopped onion
- 1 clove garlic, minced
- 1 whole small dried hot Chile pepper, seeds removed, crushed
- ¼ cup cooking oil
- salt and pepper

Instructions

Discard dandelion green roots; wash greens well in water. Cut leaves into 2-inch pieces. Cook greens uncovered in small amount of salted water until tender, about 10 minutes. Sauté onion, garlic, and chili pepper in oil. Toss and serve.

BROCCOLI RABE WITH CARAMELIZED ONIONS AND GARLIC

- 1 bunch broccoli rabe
- 2 teaspoons olive oil
- 2 large onions, cut into half moons
- 2 cloves garlic, minced
- a healthy pinch of sea salt
- freshly ground black pepper to taste

Instructions

Wash broccoli rabe well. Remove the thick part of the stems. Roughly chop.

In a large frying pan heat oil.

Add onions and sauté until they begin to brown, about 15-20 minutes.

Add garlic, broccoli rabe and sea salt. Stir-fry for about 4-5 minutes.

Add water if necessary. Make sure it remains bright green and still slightly crispy.

Variations:

Add toasted pine nuts.

Add ½ pound cooked grains to the finished greens for a light meal.

If you don't like the bitterness of broccoli rabe, blanch it before sautéing.

COLLARDS WITH DILL AND PARSLEY

- ¾ lb collard greens (6 or 7 cups, chopped)
- 2 teaspoon extra virgin olive oil
- 2 carrots, cut diagonally into ¼ inch ovals
- ½ cup water
- 2 teaspoon chopped fresh dill
- ¼ cup minced fresh parsley
- 1 tablespoon freshly squeezed lemon juice

Instructions

Wash collard greens in a large basin of cool water. Trim stalks from greens and discard. Lay several leaves one on top of the other, roll into a fat cigar shape, and slice cross-wise into 1/4-inch strips. Set aside. Repeat with remaining leaves.

Heat the oil in a large skillet. Add the carrots and cook for two minutes, stirring frequently.

Add prepared collard greens and toss to coat with the oil, about 1 minute. Add water, cover, and cook for 8-10 minutes over medium-high heat. Check tenderness of greens, and sprinkle with a pinch of salt.

Stir in dill and parsley and cook for 1 minute. Season to taste with the lemon juice and serve immediately.

SWEET VEGETABLES

Courtesy of Integrative Nutrition

There are certain vegetables, which when cooked have a deep, sweet flavor. The main ones are corn, carrots, onions, beets, winter squash and sweet potato. Then there are other less known sweet vegetables like turnip, parsnip and rutabaga. Then there are vegetables that don't taste sweet, but their effect on the body is similar to sweet vegetables. These include red radishes, daikon radish, green cabbage, red cabbage, burdock, etc.

Use two to five of the above vegetables.

Chop the hardest ones, like carrots and other roots, into smaller pieces.

Softer vegetables, like onions and cabbage, can be cut into larger chunks.

Use the layered-look. Add the vegetables into the pot in layers, so they cook evenly. Remember, the ones on the bottom will get more cooked, than the ones on the top. Add enough water to cover the bottom of the pot; 1/4 cup should be enough, just check the water level while cooking.

At the end, empty the ingredients into a large bowl and use the leftover cooking water as a delicious, sweet sauce.

SPICY KALE-ALMOND PESTO AND CHICKPEA RATATOULI

- 1 bunch kale, washed and drained
- ½ cup whole almonds, toasted
- 1½ tablespoons garlic (about 5 large cloves)
- 1/8 teaspoon salt
- ¼ to ½ teaspoon crushed red pepper flakes
- ½ teaspoon salt
- Juice of two lemons, divided
- 2 tablespoons extra-virgin olive oil
- 1 19-ounce can chickpea beans, rinsed and drained
- 1 teaspoon extra-virgin olive oil
- Freshly ground black pepper

Instructions

Cut lower stems from kale. Steam kale over 2 quarts boiling water for 5–7 minutes, until tender. Transfer to a colander to drain. Do not discard water.

Meanwhile, place almonds in a food processor and process until well chopped. Add garlic, ½ teaspoon salt, and juice of one lemon. Carefully squeeze water from steamed kale and remove leaves from stems; discard stems. Pat leaves dry with paper towels and chop roughly. Pat dry again and add to food processor. Process until all ingredients are finely minced. With motor running, add 2 tablespoons olive oil in a stream until a thick pesto is formed.

In a medium bowl, toss beans with juice of one lemon and 1/8 teaspoon salt.

In a large skillet, heat 1 teaspoon olive oil over medium heat. Add crushed red pepper flakes and fry for about 1 minute. Add kale-almond pesto and cook, stirring, for about 30 seconds. If pesto seems too thick, thin with a small amount of water. Add beans and toss gently until thoroughly heated. Sprinkle with black pepper and serve immediately.

CHINESE GREEN BEAN SALAD

- 1 pound fresh green beans
- 1 cup slivered red onion

Dressing:

- 4 teaspoons dry mustard powder
- 1 tablespoon cold water
- 1 tablespoon finely chopped fresh ginger root
- 3 tablespoons Ume plum vinegar
- 2 teaspoons dark-roasted sesame oil
- 2 teaspoonsxylitol or stevia

Instructions

Trim and cut the green beans into 1-inch lengths. Cook in rapidly boiling water, about 5 minutes or until crunchy-tender. Drain beans, immerse in cold water to stop the cooking until they are cool, then drain well.

Mix the dressing ingredients in a small bowl with a whisk until well blended.

Toss the green beans with the ginger root, red onion and dressing. Serve immediately.

ROASTED ROOT VEGETABLE AND APPLE CIDER SOUP

- 2 Dark reddish-brown sweet potatoes, yam or Japanese sweet potato
- 1 cup Parsnips, peeled and diced
- 1 cup carrots, peeled and diced
- 1 Onion- quartered
- 3 Garlic, cloves, minced
- 1 Tablespoon Fresh thyme- minced
- 1 Tablespoon Fresh sage- minced
- 1 small Butternut squash, carrot and parsnip peeled and cut into 1" pieces
- 2 Tablespoon Extra virgin olive oil
- 5 cups Chicken stock or vegetable stock
- 1-2 cups water with 2 tbsp apple cider vinegar
- 1/4 teaspoon Nutmeg
- salt and white pepper to season

Instructions

Preheat oven to 425 degrees, peel sweet potatoes, cut into dice and toss in a bowl with prepared butternut squash, parsnips, carrots garlic, onion, herbs and olive oil.

Place the mixture on a baking sheet in a single layer. Roast the vegetables for about 35 minutes or until browned evenly and caramelized. Stir vegetables as necessary to ensure even browning. Remove vegetable from the oven, puree vegetables in food processor (in batches if necessary) with a little bit of the stock if it is too thick.

Place pureed vegetables in stockpot along with the remaining water with apple cider vinegar, bring to a simmer, season with nutmeg, salt and pepper as necessary. Cook mixture for about 15 minutes until it is heated through. If soup is too thick adjust by adding extra stock or more cider. Garnish with Almond or Cashew Butter and a little extra nutmeg if desired.

ITALIAN-STYLE GARBANZO BEANS

- 1 tablespoon olive oil
- 2 cans 19-oz garbanzo beans (chickpeas), drained
- 1 can 14 ½-oz salt-free stewed chopped tomatoes
- 1 teaspoon chopped garlic
- 1 teaspoon ground cumin
- ½ teaspoon salt

Instructions

In a pan, combine all the ingredients; cover and bake for 15 to 20 minutes, until heated through, stirring occasionally. Serve immediately.

Fish, Fowl and Meats

ROASTED SALMON WITH STIR-FRY VEGETABLES

- 12 ounces of salmon, cut into two fillets
- ½ lemon
- 1 tablespoon coconut oil
- 2 cloves garlic (chopped)
- 1 tablespoon fresh ginger (grated)
- ¼ cup onions (chopped)
- 2 cups cherry tomatoes, halved
- 5 oz. can of water chestnuts, drained
- 3 cups baby spinach leaves, steamed

Instructions

Preheat oven to 350 degrees.

Rinse the salmon well and rub with lemon juice. Place the fillets on a cake rack, laid on a cookie sheet, on the middle rack of the oven. You can place the fillets directly on the cookie sheet, but raising them keeps the fish a little firmer. Bake for 20 minutes.

While the salmon is cooking, heat the oil in a frying pan and add the garlic, onion and ginger. Stir fry for 2 minutes. Add the tomatoes and water chestnuts, fry until heated through and fold in the steamed spinach. Serve alongside the salmon.

LIME-BAKED FISH

- ½ lb. fresh fish fillets
- ¼ cup fresh lime juice
- 1 teaspoon tarragon leaves
- ¼ cup chopped green onion tops

Instructions

Arrange the fish fillets in a baking dish. Sprinkle with the lime juice, tarragon, and onion tops. Bake, covered, at 325°F for 15–20 minutes or until the fish flakes easily.

ORANGE ROUGHY IN SCALLION AND GINGER SAUCE

- 2 teaspoons sesame oil
- ¼ cup finely chopped green onion
- 1 teaspoon freshly grated ginger
- 1 teaspoon finely chopped garlic
- 2 orange roughy fillets

Instructions

Preheat the oven to 400°F. Mix the sesame oil, onion, ginger, and garlic in a small bowl. Place the fish fillets in an ovenproof casserole dish. Drizzle the marinade over the fish and bake for 12 minutes or until the fish flakes easily.

Cod, sole, or flounder may be substituted for the orange roughy.

SNAPPER VERA CRUZ

- 2 red snapper fillets (¾-inch thick), no skin
- ½ medium red onion, chopped
- ½ teaspoon Serrano chili pepper, minced
- 2 2/3 tablespoons sliced ripe green olives
- 1 tablespoon chopped fresh cilantro, if desired
- 1 tablespoons tomato paste
- 1 ½ tablespoons extra virgin olive oil
- 1 cloves garlic, minced
- ½ teaspoon green pepper, minced
- Olive oil cooking spray

Instructions

Coat a large nonstick skillet and a 11 x 7 x 2 inch baking dish with the Olive oil cooking spray. Place the red snapper fillets in the baking dish. On low heat sauté the onions, garlic, and extra virgin olive oil for about 4 minutes, add the Mexican oregano, Chablis wine, green olives, red onion, tomato paste, chili pepper, and green pepper; bring to a boil and simmer until it has thickened (10 – 15 minutes). Pour over fillets and bake at 400°F for about 25 minutes, until fish flakes easily. Garnish with the cilantro sprigs, if desired.

BROILED SOLE IN LEMON SAUCE

- 1 ½ tablespoons olive oil or ghee or butter
- ½ cup lemon juice
- 2 sole fillets

Instructions

Place the spread or spray in a medium saucepan. Whisk in the lemon juice, bring it to a boil and reduce the sauce slightly. Stir in the half-and-half and keep warm.

Meanwhile, preheat the broiler and place the fish on an unheated rack in a broiler pan. Broil 4"–6" from the heat and cook for 2–6 minutes or until it flakes easily. Remove the fish to a serving platter and spoon the sauce over the fish.

BAKED HALIBUT WITH SALSA VERDE

- 1 ½ pounds halibut steak
- 1 teaspoon olive oil, preferably extra-virgin

Salsa verde

- 1 ½ tablespoons olive oil, preferably extra-virgin
- 1 tablespoon minced shallots
- 1 small clove garlic, minced
- Salt and freshly ground black pepper to taste
- 2 tablespoons very finely chopped fresh cilantro or a Italian flat leaf parsley
- 1 teaspoon fresh lemon juice
- 1 teaspoon almond butter

Instructions

To bake halibut:

Preheat oven to 300°F. Set halibut on a large sheet of aluminum foil, drizzle with oil and season with salt and pepper. Bring together sides and ends of foil and seal into a tent, leaving an air space on top. Transfer tent to a large baking dish or baking sheet. Bake until the interior of the fish is opaque, 15 to 20 minutes.

To make salsa verde:

Combine oil, parsley, shallots, capers, garlic, lemon juice and almond in a small bowl. Season with salt and pepper.

Divide baked halibut into 4 medallions. Spoon a little salsa verde on top of each portion and serve.

CHERRY SNAPPER CEVICHE

- 2 cherry snapper (tilapia) fillets, medium diced
- juice of 1 ½ fresh limes
- ¼ teaspoon red chili garlic paste (or finely ground garlic and red pepper paste)
- 1 ripe Roma tomato, medium diced
- ¼ small yellow Spanish onion, medium diced
- 1 ½ tablespoon fresh cilantro, finely chopped
- Kosher salt
- black pepper

Instructions

Soak the diced fish in ¾ of the lime juice for 3 hours. Drain off the liquid and discard.

Mix the fish with the red chili garlic paste, tomatoes, onion, cilantro, and the remaining lime juice. Season with salt and pepper. The fish is cooked by the lime's acidity rather than by the heat.

CHICKEN MOLE

- 1 ¼ pounds chicken breast tenders
- ½ large onion, chopped
- ½ large green bell pepper, cored, seeded, and chopped
- ½ cloves garlic, minced
- 1 tablespoon chili powder
- ¼ teaspoon ground cinnamon
- Salt
- Ground black pepper
- ¼ teaspoon ground cloves
- ½ can (7 ¼ oz.) diced tomatoes
- 1 tablespoon unsweetened natural almond butter
- 1 tablespoon unsweetened, cocoa powder
- 1 scallion, chopped

Instructions

Sprinkle the chicken with salt and black pepper. Heat a large nonstick skillet coated with olive oil cooking spray over medium-high heat. Add the chicken and cook for 8 minutes, turning once, or until browned on both sides. Remove the chicken to a large plate.

Add the onion, bell pepper, and garlic to the skillet and cook for 3 minutes, or until the onion becomes translucent. Stir in the chili powder, cinnamon, and cloves and cook for 1 minute. Return the chicken to the skillet. Add the tomatoes (with juice), almond butter, and cocoa powder and bring to a boil. Cover and simmer, stirring every few minutes, for 25 minutes, turning once, or until the chicken is no longer pink. Garnish with the scallions.

HERB-MARINATED CHICKEN

- 2 boneless, skinless chicken breast halves
- 2/3 tablespoon extra-virgin olive oil or coconut oil
- 1/3 tablespoon lemon juice
- 2/3 teaspoon dried crushed basil
- 1/3 teaspoon dried crushed oregano or tarragon
- dash onion powder
- 2/3 cloves garlic, minced

Instructions

Set a heavy zip-top food-storage bag in a large mixing bowl and place the Chicken in the bag. Add the oil, Ume plum vinegar, basil, oregano or tarragon, onion powder, and garlic. Close the bag and turn it to coat the chicken well. Marinate for 5–24 hours in the refrigerator, turning occasionally.

Drain the chicken, reserving the marinade. Place the chicken on an unheated rack in a broiler pan. Brush with the marinade. Broil 4"–5" from the heat for about 20 minutes or until lightly browned, brushing often with the marinade. Turn the chicken and broil for 5–15 minutes more, until the chicken is tender and no longer pink.

WALNUT CHICKEN BREAST STIR FRY

- 2 chicken breasts, skinless, boneless
- 2 tablespoons walnut oil
- ¼ teaspoon ground ginger
- ½ medium onion
- ¼ cup chicken broth
- 2 cups broccoli flowerettes
- ½ red bell pepper
- ¼ cup chopped walnuts
- ¼ teaspoon garlic, minced
- ½ green bell pepper
- 2 cups assorted greens

Instructions

In a large bowl, combine 1 tablespoon walnut oil and ground ginger. Set aside. Cut the peppers and onion into 1 inch pieces. Cut the chicken breasts into 1 inch pieces. Add the chicken to the large bowl, stir to coat. Cover, then place in the refrigerator for 30 minutes.

While waiting; in a small bowl combine the ginger with the reduced sodium chicken broth. Set aside.

In a large skillet (or Wok), heat the remaining walnut oil over medium high-heat, when hot, but not smoking, add the chicken (discard all remaining marinade), cook until chicken is no longer pink. Remove chicken, set aside. Now stir fry the onion and peppers until onion is tender, add the broccoli, cook until tender, add chicken and broth mixture, cook stirring constantly until chicken is brought up to desired serving temperature. Turn off heat, add walnuts, and stir thoroughly. On 2 serving plates, divide the mixed greens evenly, and then pour walnut chicken mixture onto center of greens.

CHICKEN PICCATA

- ¾ pound whole skinless boneless chicken breast, halved lengthwise
- 1 tablespoon extra virgin olive oil
- 2 tablespoons ghee or butter
- ¼ teaspoon paprika
- 2 tablespoons minced fresh parsley
- 1 tablespoon lemon juice
- Salt and pepper to taste

Instructions

Pound the chicken pieces to flatten them slightly. Season them with salt and pepper to taste. Heat an empty pan on high heat, then add the oil and one tablespoon of the butter and allow that to get hot (but not smoking). Then carefully add the chicken, making sure the oil doesn't splatter. Doing this process will prevent the chicken from sticking. If you heat the oil and pan together, or if the pan isn't hot enough, the chicken will stick. Sauté the chicken pieces for 1 minute on each side, or until they are cooked through. Transfer the chicken with tongs to a platter and cover it loosely to keep it warm.

Pour off any remaining fat and oil from the skillet. Return it to the stovetop and add the remaining 1 tablespoon ghee and the lemon juice, and bring the mixture to a boil. Stir in the capers, the parsley, the paprika, and salt and pepper to taste, and spoon the sauce over the chicken. Serve with 1 cup wilted spinach per person.

CHIPOTLE CHICKEN AND BUTTERNUT SQUASH SOUP

- 1 (7-ounce) can chipotle chiles in adobo sauce
- 1 tablespoon olive oil
- 1 cup red bell pepper, diced small
- ¼ yellow onion, chopped fine
- 1 tablespoon minced garlic
- 1 tablespoon dried thyme
- 2 tablespoons fresh parsley, chopped fine
- 1 teaspoon ground cumin
- 2 boneless chicken breasts
- 2 (14 ½-ounce) cans chicken stock
- 1 (14 ½-ounce) can diced tomatoes
- 1 Diced butternut squash
- Chopped green onions (for garnish, optional)

Instructions

Saute butternut squash in fry pan with ½ tablespoon olive oil then add ½ cup water to steam until squash is soft. Remove squash to soup pot. Dice chicken into bite-size pieces. Toss with salt, pepper, cumin, and thyme. Remove 1 chipotle Chile from can (reserve the remaining Chiles and sauce for another use) and puree with chickpeas and parsley in food processor until smooth. Add enough chicken stock to make a thick but spreadable paste.

Heat the oil in a large saucepan over medium-high heat and sauté bell pepper, onions, and garlic, about 5 minutes. Add seasoned chicken and continue to cook, stirring to sear chicken on all sides, about 3 minutes. Stir in squash and cook just until it becomes aromatic. Add canned tomatoes and additional chicken stock to your preferred thickness. Bring to a boil for just a minute, and then reduce to a simmer for at least another 5 to 10 minutes to let the flavors mix and develop. Season to taste. Top each serving with a pinch of green onions.

Grains

For all grain recipes, it is best to soak the grain in water with a teaspoon or two of Ume plum vinegar or lemon juice. The longer you soak the grain the better; you can even soak them over night. Drain the grain and then add water (2 to 1 water to grain in most instances).

ZESTY QUINOA WITH BROCCOLI & CASHEWS

- ½ tablespoon extra virgin olive oil
- 1 cloves garlic, minced
- ¼ medium red onion, finely diced
- ¼ cup sun-dried tomatoes, julienned or chopped
- ¼ cup vegetable broth
- 1 tablespoon lemon juice
- ¼ cup quinoa
- ¼ teaspoon sea salt, or to taste
- ½ cup broccoli cut into bite-sized pieces Fresh ground black pepper to taste
- ¼ cup roasted cashew pieces
- 1 scallions, thinly sliced

Instructions

Heat the olive oil over medium heat in a saucepan and sauté the onion and garlic for 3 minutes. Add the sun-dried tomatoes, vegetable stock, wine and lemon juice and bring to a boil.

Stir in the quinoa and salt. Reduce heat, and simmer covered about 20 minutes. Add the broccoli on top and simmer an additional 5 to 6 minutes.

Remove from heat, toss gently until combined. Add ground pepper and additional salt, if desired, to taste. Garnish with cashews and scallions before serving.

BAKED STUFFED PEPPERS

- ½ cup long-grain brown rice
- Salt to taste
- 4 large red or green sweet peppers
- 3 tablespoon butter or ghee
- 1 medium onion, chopped
- ½ cup finely diced celery

- ½ cup sunflower seeds
- ¼ cup minced parsley
- ¼ teaspoon dried oregano leaves, crumbled
- ¼ cup (4 ounces) chopped green chiles
- black pepper to taste

Instructions

Cook rice in 1 ½ cups boiling salted water for 35 minutes or until tender. Drain if necessary. Set aside.

Cut peppers in half. Remove seeds and white membrane. Parboil peppers in boiling salted water for 5 minutes. Arrange in slightly oiled, shallow 1-½ quart baking dish.

Melt butter in small skillet. Add onion, celery, and sunflower seeds. Sauté until onion is tender. Remove from heat. Stir into rice. Add parsley, oregano, chiles, black pepper, and salt to taste. Fill peppers with mixture. Put about 1/3 cup hot water in bottom of dish. Bake at 400 degrees for about 20 minutes.

CHICKEN & RICE

- 2 cups brown rice (soak for 30 minutes)
- 2 tablespoon olive oil
- 1/2 lb skinless, boneless chicken (cut into small cubes)
- 1 med. onion (chopped)
- 4 cloves garlic (minced)
- ¼ cup lemon juice
- 2 cups simmering chicken stock
- 1/4 teaspoon ground black pepper
- 1/2 cup butter

Instructions

Heat the olive oil. Add the chicken cubes and cook, stirring until they start to turn white. Sauté the garlic, oil. Stir in the rice. Sauté for two minutes. Add the lemon juice and bring to a boil. Simmer gently until almost all the wine is absorbed. Add the simmering stock and cook until the rice is just tender. Add the butter and stir well. Season with sea salt and black pepper. Serve hot.

BROWN RICE WITH MIX VEGETABLES

- 2 cups brown rice (soak for 30 minutes)
- ½ cup celery (diced)
- 1 med. onion (chopped)
- 4 cloves garlic (minced)
- 1 cup carrots (diced)
- 4 tablespoon olive oil
- 3 cups simmering chicken stock

Instructions

In a pan, heat the olive oil. Sauté the garlic, onion and the vegetable. Stir in the rice. Sauté for two minutes. Add the simmering stock and let boil before turning the flame to low. Cook until the rice is done. Best served with fish, chicken or meat.

BROWN RICE CASSEROLE

- 4 cups cooked brown rice
- ½ cup chopped parsley
- ½ cup slivered olives
- ½ cup butter
- 2 tablespoon fish sauce (asian section of grocery store)
- ½ teaspoon ground black pepper

Instructions

In a wok, heat the butter. Add the olives, parsley, and rice. Mix thoroughly. Season with black pepper. Turn into prepared casserole and sprinkle paprika on top. Bake for about 30 minutes.

BROWN RICE & GREEN BELL PEPPER

- 4 cups cooked brown rice
- 4 tablespoon olive oil
- 1 cup tomato puree or sauce
- 2 tablespoon fish sauce
- 2 med. green bell pepper (squares)
- 1 med. onion (chopped)
- ¼ teaspoon ground black pepper

Instructions

Heat oil in a pan. Sauté onion and green bell pepper. Add the tomato sauce. Season with fish sauce and black pepper. Mix the cooked rice thoroughly. Serve while hot. This is best eaten with chicken, pork or beef.

SAVORY BROWN RICE

- 4 cups cooked brown rice
- 1 cup thinly sliced mushrooms
- 1 teaspoon lemon juice
- 4 tablespoon butter
- 1 med. onion (chopped)

Instructions

In a pan, heat the butter and sauté the onion. Add the mushrooms. Mix the cooked brown rice. Season with sea salt. This is best served with burger steak, fish steak or chicken.

FRIED BROWN RICE

- 1 and ½ cup leftover brown rice
- 1 tablespoon carrot, diced
- ¼ cabbage, cut into strips
- ¼ leftover meat, diced
- 1 teaspoon cooking oil
- ¼ teaspoon red paprika powder
- 1 teaspoon sea salt to taste

Instructions

Cooking brown rice (if no leftover rice is available)

Measure 1 c of brown rice into cooking utensil. Brown rice may be cooked using a rice cooker or pot. Add 2 c water to the brown rice. Let stand for 30 minutes to soak. If using rice cooker, leave the cooker undisturbed for 15 minutes. Continue cooking for 20 minutes. For best results, leave the cooked rice undisturbed for 15 minutes.

Cooking of fried rice

Heat cooking oil in a skillet. Stir fry meat, carrot and cabbage for 2 minutes. Add spices mix and stir well. Combine brown rice with the mixture and continue cooking for 5 minutes with constant stirring. Season with salt

QUINOA PORRIDGE

- ½ cup quinoa
- ½ cup berries
- xylitol or stevia optional
- 1 teaspoon ghee
- cinnamon to taste
- Toasted almonds optional

Instructions

Cook quinoa and while hot chop up the berries and kind of mash it into the mixture then let margarine melt and add cinnamon, nuts and sweeteners if desired. It's really warming and satisfying!

QUINOA STUFFING

Quinoa:

- 2 Tablespoons minced onion
- 2 Tablespoons butter
- 1 ½ cups quinoa
- About 4 cups veggie or chicken stock, warmed

Stuffing:

- 2 cloves garlic
- 2 large onion, medium dice
- 2 carrots, medium dice
- 2 celery stalks, medium dice
- 1/3 cup olive oil
- ¼ cup flax seed
- 3 cups cooked quinoa (recipe follows)
- ¼ cup fresh thyme, picked

Instructions

For quinoa:

Melt butter in a pot over medium heat. Gently sweat onions until translucent. Add quinoa and toast slightly for about a minute. Add ½ cup seasoned stock and simmer until quinoa absorbs the liquid. Keep adding stock a little at a time until the quinoa grain opens. When it opens, a small tail-like pistol will pop out. It should be tender to the bite. Remove quinoa from pot and cool on sheet tray. Check seasonings and adjust if necessary. If the stock was well seasoned, the quinoa should not need any further seasoning.

For stuffing:

Preheat oven to 375°F. Heat olive oil in large pot over medium heat. Sweat garlic, onions, carrots andcelery until tender. Season with a pinch of salt. Add cooked quinoa and thyme; toss to bind. Add stock to moisten to liking. Transfer to baking dish and bake, uncovered for 45 minutes.

CRUNCHY QUINOA SALAD

Dressing:

- 6 tablespoon olive oil
- 1 tablespoon lemon juice
- 1 ½ teaspoon black pepper

Salad:

- 1 cup quinoa, rinsed well
- 1 ¾ cups cool water
- ¼ lb. carrots, shredded/grated
- ¼ cup sesame seeds
- ¼ cup sunflower seeds
- 3 stalks green onion
- ¼ bunch parsley chopped fine

Instructions

Cook quinoa till water is absorbed. Cooking time can vary from 25-45 minutes; just keep an eye on it, and stir several times during cooking process. While quinoa is cooking, make dressing by mixing together all dressing ingredients. After quinoa is cooked, mix it with all other salad ingredients. Coat with dressing.

Mix thoroughly.

You can serve it warm or chilled.

AMARANTH WITH SPINACH TOMATO SAUCE

- 1 cup amaranth seed
- 2 ½ cups water
- 1 Tablespoon olive oil
- 1 bunch spinach
- 2 ripe tomatoes, skinned and coarsely chopped
- 1 teaspoon basil
- 1 teaspoon oregano
- 1 clove of garlic minced
- 1 tablespoon onion, minced
- Sea salt and pepper to taste (or use a salt substitute)

Instructions

Add amaranth to boiling water, bring back to boil, reduce heat, cover and simmer for 18-20 minutes.

While amaranth is cooking, stem and wash spinach, then simmer until tender. Dip tomatoes into boiling water to loosen skin, then peel and chop. Heat oil in a skillet over medium heat and add garlic an onion. Sauté approximately 2 minutes. Add tomato, basil, oregano, salt, pepper and 1 tablespoon of water. Drain and chop spinach and add to tomato mixture. Cook an addition 10 to15 minutes, stirring occasionally. Lightly mash tomato as it is cooking.

Stir the sauce into the amaranth or spoon it on top.

AMARANTH "GRITS"

- 1 cup amaranth
- 1 clove garlic, finely chopped or pressed
- 1 medium onion, finely chopped
- 3 cups water or vegetable stock
- Sea salt to taste
- Garnish: 2 plum tomatoes

Instructions

Combine the amaranth, garlic, onion, and stock in a 2-quart saucepan. Boil; reduce heat and simmer covered until most of the liquid has been absorbed, about 20 minutes. Stir well. If the mixture is too thin or the amaranth not quite tender (it should be crunchy, but not gritty hard), boil gently while stirring constantly until thickened, about 30 seconds. Add salt to taste. Stir in a few drops of hot sauce, if desired, and garnish with chopped tomatoes.

QUINOA OR AMARANTH TABOULI

- 1 cup quinoa or amaranth
- 1 cup parsley, chopped
- ½ cup scallions, chopped
- 2 tablespoon fresh mint
- ½ cup lemon juice
- ¼ cup olive oil
- 2 garlic cloves, pressed
- ¼ cup olives, sliced

Instructions

Simmer quinoa or amaranth in an equal volume of water for 12-15 minutes. Allow to cool.

Place all ingredients except lettuce and olives in a mixing bowl and toss together lightly. Chill for an hour or more to allow flavors to blend.

AMARANTH OR QUINOA PUDDING

- 2 cups amaranth or quinoa, cooked
- ½ cup almonds, chopped fine
- 1 ½ teaspoon vanilla
- ½ tablespoon xylitol or stevia
- 1 cup water
- juice of ½ lemon
- grated rind of one lemon
- dash of cinnamon

Instructions

Combine ingredients in a large sauce pan, cover and bring to a boil. Reduce heat and simmer for 15 minutes. Pour pudding into individual dessert bowls. Top with a few strawberries and chill.

AMARANTH OR QUINOA STIR-FRY

- 2 cups cooked amaranth or quinoa
- 2 Tablespoon oil
- 1 onion, chopped
- 1 carrot, sliced
- 1 celery stalk, sliced
- 3 cloves garlic, chopped fine
- ½ cup almonds, chopped
- ¼ cup sunflower seeds
- 1 teaspoon sea salt

Instructions

Sauté veggies, garlic, almonds and seeds in the oil until vegetables are tender crisp. Add seasonings and amaranth or quinoa. Mix well until warmed through

QUINOA CILANTRO TABBOULEH

- 2 cups water
- 1 cup quinoa
- 3 Tablespoon extra virgin olive oil
- 3 cloves garlic
- ¼ cup lemon juice
- ½ cup scallions, minced
- ¾ cup fresh cilantro, chopped
- ¼ cup pine nuts

Instructions

Bring water to a boil over high heat. Add quinoa, reduce heat to low and cover. Cook 15-20 minutes, until water is absorbed and kernels are soft. Transfer to a bowl and refrigerate. Combine oil, garlic, lemon juice and sea salt to taste in a jar with a tight fitting lid. Shake well and combine with remaining ingredients, except salad greens. Stir in quinoa and chill. Serve!

MILLET SALAD

- 2 cups millet, soaked overnight, rinsed and drained
- handful or two of fresh picked cilantro
- 4 green onions, sliced thin
- 1 large carrot, shredded
- ½ cucumber, diced
- 2 tablespoon mustard powder
- 2 Tablespoon Ume plum vinegar
- ¾ cup organic olive oil
- sea salt to taste

Instructions

Place soaked, rinsed millet in a saucepan on the stove and add the same amount of water by volume. Add in a couple of pinches of sea salt and put the heat on medium-high. Once the pot is boiling, turn it down to a simmer.

Once all the water has absorbed (about 15 minutes), remove from heat to let cool. Add a little bit of olive oil and fluff the millet with a fork, just to keep it from sticking together (or to separate it if it already has stuck). You want the millet to cool to room temperature, so if you want to hurry it along, you might want to transfer it to a bowl.

While millet is cooling you can prepare the dressing. Mix mustard powder and Ume plum vinegar in a bowl with a pinch of salt. Using a whisk, mix mixture vigorously while adding in the olive oil in a thin stream. The dressing will thicken as you add more oil. Once all oil has been incorporated you can stop whisking. Set aside.

Combine cucumber, carrot, green onion, and cilantro with the cooled millet and stir. Pour dressing over millet mixture and stir well. Add more salt if necessary.

SPINACH SALAD WITH WARM QUINOA

- 1 5-oz. container of baby spinach
- 1 cup quinoa, soaked overnight, drained and rinsed
- 2 green onions, diced
- handful of cherry tomatoes, halved
- 1 tablespoon organic butter
- pinch of sea salt
- 2 tablespoon tahini
- ½ a cucumber, sliced
- handful of shelled sunflower seeds

Instructions

Pour a tablespoon or so of olive oil into a medium sized saucepan that's been heated on the stove-top. Add in strained quinoa, stirring frequently while it toasts in the bottom of the pot.

Once you get a whiff of that toasted quinoa, it's probably time to add the water. Add a cup of water and sea salt, cover the pot and bring it to a boil. Once it's boiled turn it down to a simmer. Simmer the quinoa for 15 or 20 minutes, or until all the water has soaked up and the grains are tender. Remove from heat and let cool for ten minutes.

While quinoa is cooling, toss spinach, green onion, cucumber, sunflower seeds and tomato in a large bowl. Spoon in the 2 tablespoon tahini in dabs and toss well. Add warm quinoa and toss yet again, allowing the spinach to wilt a little. Pour over dressing your dressing of choice and mix.

The Cleanse Advanced Recipes

GAGA GOOD SHAKE

- 1 green apple
- ½ cucumber
- 1 lime (peeled)
- 2 cups fresh spinach
- 1 avocado
- 1 teaspoon stevia or xylitol

Instructions

Blend on high speed adding water as need to the desired texture. Serve immediately.

Variations:

Add coconut milk or fresh almond milk for a creamier shake

Add 1 tablespoon fresh grated ginger

THE RAW SALAD SMASH

- 1 bunch of kale
- 1 whole head of celery
- 1 lemon
- 1 handful of spinach leaves
- 1 avocado
- 1 teaspoon lemon-lime Greens Powder
- 1 chili pepper

Instructions

Put kale, celery and lemon through juicer or blender adding water as need to the desired texture. Then combine in blender with remaining ingredients.

RAW-TASTIC V8 JUICE

- 1 medium-sized carrots
- ¼ bag baby spinach
- ¼ red bell pepper
- 1 stalks celery
- ½ clove garlic
- 1 large tomatoes
- ¼ head fresh cabbage
- ¼ green bell pepper
- 1-2 kale leaves
- chili pepper to taste
- salt to taste

Instructions

Run all the vegetables through your juicer or blender, adding water as need to the desired texture and add salt to taste. Any hot sauce can be substituted for chili pepper.

MINT MADNESS

- ½ cucumbers
- juice of 1 lime
- juice of 1 lemon
- 1 avocado
- 1 cup raw spinach
- ½ can coconut milk
- 2-4 springs for fresh mint leaves
- ice

Instructions

Combine all ingredients and blend. adding water as need to the desired texture.

VEGGIE-VENGENCE SHAKE

- ¼ cup flax seed oil or olive oil
- 2 small cucumbers
- 1 cup spinach
- ½ cup broccoli
- ¼ cup cilantro
- ½ medium tomato
- ¼ cup parsley
- 2 stalks celery, cut into pieces
- 1/8 cup fresh cilantro leaves
- 2 medium limes (or 1 lemon)
- 1/8 cup fresh dill (optional)
- 1 cup water

Instructions

Place water in a blender then add oil. Turn blender on low speed and add remaining ingredients one at a time. When everything is chopped up, turn blender to high speed until you get a beautiful smooth and creamy shake.

Soups

SIMPLE GREEN GAZPACHO SOUP

- 1 cucumber, cubed
- 1 zucchini, cubed
- 1 avocado, cubed
- mint (optional)

Instructions

Place ingredients in a blender adding water as need to the desired texture. Mix until almost smooth. Serve garnished with mint leaf.

CLASSIC GAZPACHO

- 4 cups fresh tomato juice or canned in a pinch
- ½ cup cucumber, chopped
- ¼ cup green bell pepper, chopped
- ¼ cup celery, finely chopped
- 1 Tbs olive oil
- ½ teaspoon pepper
- 5 leaves basil
- ½ teaspoon garlic, minced

Instructions

Combine all ingredients. Cover and chill overnight.

PROVENCE PUREE

- 1 avocado
- 2 stalks celery
- 1 head Romaine lettuce
- 1 small tomato
- 1 handful spinach
- 1 small cucumber, peeled
- 2 cloves garlic
- 1/3 onion
- 2 tablespoons olive oil
- herbes de provence

Instructions

Puree all vegetables with a juicer or blender with a blank blade for pureeing, doing the onion last. Mix in olive oil, and herbes du Provence to taste. Serve with sprouts sprinkled on top.

MEAN JOE GREEN GAZPACHO

- 2 avocados
- 1 head Romaine lettuce
- 3 cloves garlic
- ¼ cup fresh lemon juice
- ¼ teaspoon sea salt
- 2 tablespoons olive oil
- 2 green bell pepper
- 6 roma tomatoes
- 1 large cucumbers
- ½ red onion
- 1 teaspoons basil
- ½ teaspoon dill
- ½ teaspoon oregano

Instructions

Chop all vegetables. Mix avocado, lemon juice and garlic in food processor (with S blade), until smooth and empty into bowl. Process tomatoes and romaine until smooth, and add to bowl. Pulse peppers, cucumbers and onion until chunky (approximately 1/8-1/4 inch) and empty into bowl. Mix well with salt and olive oil, and herbs if desired.

DREAMIN' GREEN SOUP

- 1-2 avocados
- 1-2 cucumbers, peeled and seeded
- 1 jalapeno pepper, seeded
- ½ white onion, diced
- juice of ½ lemon
- 1-2 cups vegetable stock or water
- 3 cloves roasted garlic
- 1 tablespoon fresh cilantro
- 1 tablespoon fresh parsley
- 1 carrot, finely diced

Instructions

Purée all ingredients (except onions and carrots) in a food processor or blender. Add more or less water to desired consistency. Add onions and raw crunch bits at the end for a garnish. Yum!

PREBIOTIC SOUP

- 2-3 whole garlic cloves
- 1 large onion
- 2 tablespoon fresh cilantro
- 2 tsp fresh grated ginger
- 2-3 quarts veggie broth
- 1 Jerusalem artichoke chopped (Optional: carrots, cucumber, celery and any other veggie desired)
- sea salt to taste

Instructions

Chop and crush garlic cloves into small diced pieces and lightly steam-fry. Set aside. Put whole onion in water in a deep pan, simmer until onion is transparent. Add garlic and vegetable broth. Chop Jerusalem artichoke and optional veggies) and add to soup. Simmer 10-15 minutes. Add fresh ginger, cilantro and Real Salt to taste. Optional: blend with blender.

TANGO TOMATO SOUP

- 6 medium tomatoes, blended and strained (pour through a fine mesh strainer)
- ½ avocado
- ¾ cup coconut water or coconut milk
- 1 cucumber
- sea salt to taste

Instructions

Add all ingredients adding water as need to the desired texture. Blend until smooth. Warm in pan on the stove.

CAULIFLOWER, LEEK AND CELERY SOUP

- 1 onion peeled and chopped
- 1 tablespoon olive oil
- 1 whole head of celery, trimmed & chopped 1 head cauliflower, trimmed and chopped
- 4 cups vegetable stock
- 1 leek top (all whites) rinsed well and chopped
- 1 cup almond milk
- salt, pepper to taste use seasonings of choice to taste

Instructions

Steam-fry the onion and leeks in a little water in a large soup pan for about 5 minutes without browning. Pulse-chop the celery and cauliflower in the food processor until finely chopped. Add the celery and cauliflower mix to the pan and warm until tender. Add the vegetable stock, almond milk and simmer for about 15-30 minutes, or you can leave this raw and not cook at all.

Purée the soup mixture in a blender or food processor until smooth texture is achieved. Season with salt and other seasonings of choice. Serve warm or cold.

CELERY SOUP

- 4-5 stalks of celery
- 3 cups vegetable stock

Instructions

Cook celery until tenderized. Add water and broth mix. Pour all into blender. Blend 15-29 seconds. Reheat and serve. Use flax seed oil, salt, and cayenne pepper to taste.

PARSNIP AND AVOCADO SOUP

- 1 large parsnip, grated (or just cut it up if using a Vitamix)
- ½ cup water
- 1 large stalk peeled celery, cut up
- ¼ avocado
- 2 teaspoon flaxseed oil
- Squeeze of lemon juice
- ½ teaspoon sea salt

Instructions

In a blender blend parsnip and liquid until smooth. Add remaining ingredients, blend until smooth. Warm on stove.

GREEN GATOR SOUP

- 1 large cucumber
- 1 ripe avocado
- 1 clove garlic
- juice of 1 lime
- 2 cups spinach or tender greens
- ½ cup fresh cilantro
- sea salt to taste
- top with sliced celery

Instructions

Blend ingredients in food processor until creamy and smooth. Serve in pretty bowls and decorate with your favorite toppings. Can be served at room temp or warmed on stove.

KHICHADI RECIPE

Khichadi is a simple, easily digested stew traditionally used in Auyveda during a cleanse. I have updated it here with some small tweaks

- ½ cup brown basmati rice, soaked for at least ½ hour and drained
- ½ cup mung beans or lentils, soaked in water for at least 1 hour and drained
- ½ cup vegetables, such as peas, chopped kale, spinach
- 4 cups vegetable stock, chicken stock (advanced recipes)
- 2 tablespoon Ghee or Clarified butter
- 1 teaspoon cumin
- 1 medium onion, finely chopped
- 1 teaspoon chopped ginger
- 1 teaspoon garlic sautéed until golden brown
- 1 teaspoon of turmeric powder
- ¼ teaspoon of black pepper
- 1 bay leaf

Instructions

Heat ghee (clarified butter) or olive oil in a pan over moderate heat. Add cumin or coriander seeds. Then add medium onion, finely chopped, chopped ginger and garlic and sauté until golden brown. Stir in turmeric powder, black pepper and bay leaf. Add mung beans, water, vegetables, and rice. Cook for about an hour. When the beans are completely soft, add a pinch of salt. Serve this dish with ghee and chopped fresh coriander leaves.

Basic Broths

There are very few things that are as restorative to the human body as being able to rebuild with minerals, collagen containing glucosamine. These recipes can be consumed alone or used as a base for other soups.

These recipes are adaptations from *Nourishing Traditions* by Sally Fallon.

CHICKEN OR TURKEY STOCK

- 1 whole free-range chicken or 2 to 3 pounds of bony chicken parts, such as necks, backs, breastbones and wings

- 2 carrots, peeled and coarsely chopped
- 3 celery stalks, coarsely chopped
- 1 bunch parsley
- 4 quarts cold filtered water
- 2 tablespoons vinegar
- 1 large onion, coarsely chopped

Note: Farm-raised, free-range chickens are the best choice. You do not want to pick a toxic feed-lot chicken.

Instructions

If you are using a whole chicken, cut off the wings and remove the neck and the gizzards from the cavity. Cut chicken parts into several pieces. (If you are using a whole chicken, remove the neck and wings and cut them into several pieces.)

Place chicken or chicken pieces in a large crock pot with water, vinegar and all vegetables except parsley. Put it on high, then bring to a boil, and remove scum that rises to the top.

Reduce heat, cover and simmer for 8 to 12 hours. The longer you cook the stock, the richer and more flavorful it will be. About 10 minutes before finishing the stock, add parsley. This will impart additional mineral ions to the broth. I have actually added water after 12 hours and cooked a full 24 hours for unbeleiveably rich broth. If you are cooking a whole chicken, remove the meaty parts before cooking the next 12 hours.

Remove whole chicken or pieces with a slotted spoon. If you are using a whole chicken, let cool and remove chicken meat from the carcass. Reserve for other uses, such as chicken salads, enchiladas, sandwiches or curries.

Strain the stock into a large bowl and reserve in your refrigerator until the fat rises to the top and congeals. Skim off this fat and reserve the stock in covered containers in your refrigerator or freezer.

BEEF STOCK

- 4 pounds beef marrow and knuckle bones (from local butcher)
- ½ cup vinegar
- 3 pounds meaty bones
- 4 or more quarts cold filtered water
- 3 onions, coarsely chopped
- 3 carrots, coarsely chopped
- 1 teaspoon dried green peppercorns, crushed
- 3 celery stalks, coarsely chopped
- Several sprigs of fresh thyme, tied together
- 1 bunch parsley

Instructions

Place the marrow bones in a large crock pot with vinegar and cover with water. Let stand for one hour. Meanwhile, place the meaty bones in a roasting pan and brown at 350 degrees in the oven. When well browned, add to the crock pot along with the vegetables. Pour the fat out of the roasting pan, add cold water to the pan, set over a high flame and bring to a boil, stirring with a wooden spoon to loosen up coagulated juices. Add this liquid to the crock pot.

Add additional water, if necessary, to cover the bones; but the liquid should come no higher than within one inch of the rim of the pot, as the volume expands slightly during cooking. Bring to high heat obtaining a boil. A large amount of scum will come to the top, and it is important to remove this with a spoon. After you have skimmed, reduce heat and add the thyme and crushed peppercorns.

Simmer stock for at least 12 and as long as 72 hours. Just before finishing, add the parsley and simmer another 10 minutes. You will now have a pot of brown liquid containing globs of gelatinous and fatty material.

Remove bones with tongs or a slotted spoon. Strain the stock into a large bowl. Let cool in the refrigerator and remove the congealed fat that rises to the top. Transfer to smaller containers and to the freezer for long-term storage.

CPSIA information can be obtained at www.ICGtesting.com
Printed in the USA
BVOW031114120413

318028BV00002B/6/P